MAKING USE OF BEHAVIORAL PSYCHOLOGY

How I got RID OF

MIGRAINE HEADACHES

IN 30 DAYS

With

I0424887

AROMA-CONDITIONING:

Easy Self-Help Treatment Combining

Classical Conditioning & Aromatherapy

KALIN NACHEFF

How I Got Rid of Migraine Headaches in 30 Days with Aroma-Conditioning: Easy Self-Help Treatment Combining Classical Conditioning & Aromatherapy

Printed in the United States of America

ISBN 978-1450566605

Medical Limit of Liability: The information in this book is intended to provide accurate and helpful health information for the general public. It is sold with the understanding that the author and publisher are not engaged in rendering medical, health, psychological, or any other personal professional advice. The information should not be considered as complete and does not address all medical conditions and treatments. It should not be used in place of a visit to a medical or other qualified health professional who should be consulted before using any suggestions from this book or inferring anything from it. If an individual is under a doctor or other qualified health professional's care and receives advice contrary to information provided in this book, the doctor or qualified health professional's advice should be followed, as the advice is based on the unique characteristics of that individual.

Limit of Liability/Disclaimer of Warranty: While the author and publisher have made their best efforts in preparing this book, they make no representations or warranties with respect to the accuracy or completeness of the contents of this book and specifically disclaim any implied warranties or merchantability or fitness for a particular purpose. No warranty may be created or extended by sales representatives or written sales materials. The author and publisher shall not be liable for any loss of profit or any other commercial damages, including but not limited to special, incidental, consequential, or other damages.

Designed and Illustrated by Kalin Nacheff

For more information and technical support, please contact the author:

kalin.nachev3@gmail.com

AUTHOR'S NOTE

To People with Migraines

This book includes a quick migraine guide but its main focus is on aroma-conditioning, a self-help therapy that may help you become drug-free and headache-free. The therapy is easy because after reading this book, it will take only a minute of your day to try it; aroma-conditioning doesn't require any special training—a desire to get rid of migraines and to apply simple techniques is enough. While reading about the basics of aroma-conditioning, you will learn interesting things about psychology, learning, and how the natural learning process can be as effective or even better in healing than pharmacological drugs.

Because aroma-conditioning is founded on classical conditioning, it should also be effective for the more common tension-type headaches.

The most valuable lesson I learned from my long experience with migraine headaches is that *you* have to take charge of your treatment if you want to start living a normal life. No one will be able to help you if you aren't willing to help yourself. Taking charge of your treatment mostly involves educating yourself about migraine.

To Researchers and Health-Care Professionals

The situations in this book come from my own experience. But the conclusions are based on scientific facts and established theories in psychology. I welcome all opinions based on scientific criticism.

Parts of the book resemble the layout of a research study in behavioral psychology and clinical therapy. I used that layout to make it easier for clinical and health professionals to assess my successful therapy, draw conclusions, and use my experience to help people with migraine.

Sincerely,

K. Nachaff

ABOUT THE AUTHOR

Kalin Nacheff, the author of *How I Got Rid of Migraine Headaches in 30 Days with Aroma-Conditioning* has a lifelong personal experience with migraine, being a chronic migraine sufferer himself. Nevertheless, one of his greatest achievements is getting rid of chronic migraine headaches, using the science of psychology creatively. Kalin's main reason for writing this book is his belief that aroma-conditioning will help other people with migraine lead more fulfilling lives.

Kalin Nacheff works as a freelance writer and has written articles and provided content for various companies, including leading media companies like Internet Brands, INC. His style, as an author, involves creating illustrations, cartoons, photography, photo collages and other visuals. He provides content and manages the social media accounts of Leatherup.com—the most popular online motorcycle store. He lives with his wife, Snezhana Nacheff, in Pasadena, CA.

CONTENTS

CHAPTER II

MIGRAINE: MORE THAN A HEADACHE.......19

CHAPTER III

MIGRAINES, DRUGS, AND AROMATHERAPY...26

CHAPTER IV

AROMA-CONDITIONING IN ACTION.............39

CHAPTER V

ANATOMY OF AROMA-CONDITIONING 54

CHAPTER VI

THE MAN WITH A WHITE BEARD.................62

CHAPTER VII

DRUG EFFECTS, THE RINGING BELL THEORY, AND THE MIGHTY PLACEBO.........74

CHAPTER VIII

MIGRAINE SCIENCE...............................84

HOW I GOT RID OF MIGRAINE
HEADACHES IN 30 DAYS

6:30 P.M., October 12, 1896, Imperial Institute for Experimental Medicine, St. Petersburg, Russia

A man with a white beard wearing a white coat walks into a damp, poorly lit room. He carries a can of food pellets in one hand. At the center of the room, right in front of him there's a dog bounded in leather straps and with tubes inserted in its month. A table covered with clear-glass bulbs is behind the dog. In front of the dog is some equipment. The man takes a worn, paper-covered notebook out of the pocket of his white coat. The handwritten title on the yellowish cover reads *Digestion: Experiments.* He lays the notebook and the can of food down on the table, walks to and pets the dog as he inspects and removes the tubes. He takes the can of food from the table and then crouches and hands it to the dog.

As he watches the dog eating, he remembers something. The dog was drooling before seeing the food. Wasn't it supposed to drool when the pellets were in its mouth or when it saw the pellets? The man with a white beard stands up, searching his coat pockets hastily for the pencil. He finds it behind his right ear, takes the worn notebook and starts writing out some possible tests to find the answer for what he thought was an important question.

5:00 P.M., July 12, 2006, White Oak Apartments, Pasadena, CA

A young man lies face down in bed, his skin pale, his eyes swelled, his left hand pressing a cold, moist towel against his forehead, his legs fidgeting. Though it's dark in the room, the young man uses the blanket to cover the part of his head near the window, so that the sunlight sifting through the panels of the closed shutters is blocked completely. Despite his agony, the young man is still able to think. This happened to him so many times before that it is all part of a routine: the wet towel, the dark room, and his favorite way of coping with the excruciating headache—occupying his mind with something he enjoys. Now he thinks about the man with the white beard, the dog, and the food, and then he has an interesting idea. Right then he doesn't realize that soon, his idea will free him forever from this painful condition.

The man with a white beard went on to discover the causes for the seemingly annoying drooling of the dog. In fact, he devoted the rest of his life, 30 years, to research the question. What he discovered redefined the then young science of psychology. More than 100 years later his work, which originated from his observation of a dog drooling, also inspired the young man, in the middle of a migraine attack, to find the solution to his migraine headaches. That young man was me.

Migraine Science

One hour before I lay in bed with the wet towel covering my forehead, I was preparing for a class in psychology. I had read a chapter from an introductory psychology textbook. The chapter was about learning, as understood by psychologists. I became so absorbed by this concept that I couldn't stop reading, even though my head had started throbbing with pain. What a formula, I thought. I could try to quit smoking with it. By this time, my headache had gradually become unbearable until I was unable to read. So I did what most people with migraine do. I swallowed some Advil, went to my bedroom, turned off the lights, closed the shutters, and plopped myself on the bed, hoping I would be able to make myself fall asleep.

10

In the dark room, I was left with my thoughts on the psychology of learning and the unbearable pain in my head; a mixture of pain and thoughts that led me think of an entirely new way to get rid of migraines. This idea was simple and easy to apply. And since it didn't seem to involve any health risks and was based on an established theory in the science of psychology, I decided to go along with it and experiment on myself to see if it would work. It did. I had no headaches for one year. This was my first migraine-free year as far back as I can remember.

Living in Pain

I was diagnosed with migraine headaches in early childhood and, like many people living with migraine, I ignored my condition for a long time—so long that my life was overtaken by pain.

By the end of 2003, shortly after I moved to the United States to study, the stress of living in a foreign country and of being an international student made my headaches more painful and more frequent. I had chronic daily headaches. Migraine started to affect every aspect of my life; I had headaches during college classes, commutes, and social gatherings. But I also had to work. I had to deal with customers while my head was throbbing with pain and I looked pale and sweaty. In the middle of a migraine attack my paleness made me look like a ghost, and some people who saw me at those moments thought I might be terminally ill.

At night I often woke up in pain and stayed up until the early morning hours, aching. I was trapped in a cycle of daily migraine headaches. This went on for about three years. But on that July day everything started to change.

Several months after I began my therapy, everyone around me was surprised to see me functioning normally. My colleagues at work would say, "What happen to your migraines? You haven't asked anyone lately to give you a back rub." Sometimes I would ask for a back rub if I had a headache—it would distract me from the pain. I didn't feel embarrassed to ask someone for help, because the pain was so intense. My wife's hands often became cramped because she gave me deep back massages; she couldn't bear to watch me suffer.

I was fascinated not only about what I managed to do—lead a life without headaches, but also about how I managed to do it—by applying science, creatively. After all those years of suffering, what I did to manage my migraine seemed too easy to be true. Curious, I've researched academic literature and magazines to learn more about migraine and psychology. I wanted to know everything about why and how my therapy worked. The more I learned, the more convinced I became that my experience could benefit others.

In the United States, about 30 million people live with migraine. The American Council for Headache Education (ACHE) estimated that 1 in 4 U.S. households has a person suffering from migraine (Diamond, 2007, p. 1269), which explains why migraine is among the top seven reasons for visiting a doctor (ACHE, 1994, p.1). In 2001, the World Health Organization listed migraine as one of the top 20 causes of disability.

Treating migraine can be very expensive. In the United States, the estimated per patient annual cost of migraine is $2,571, with a national burden of about $11.07 billion a year—"outpatient care, $5.21 billion; prescriptions, $4.61 billion; inpatient care, $0.73 billion; and emergency department care, $0.52 billion" (Hawkins, Rupnow & Wang, 2008, p.553).

Doctors Have Even Drilled Holes in the Skull to Try to Cure Migraines

Migraine is known as one of the most painful chronic disorders. So painful that in the past, physicians, in their attempt to find a cure went "to extremes...purging, bleeding, tying a hangman's noose around the head, applying herbs to the scalp, and even trepanning [drilling a hole in the skull] all were tried as remedies" (ACHE, 1994, p. 15). Even today, a number of "surgical procedures in and around the head and neck" are performed to treat migraine with little success (ACHE, 1994, p. 15).

No extremes were involved in the way I managed my migraines (the only extreme was coming up with a migraine therapy after studying for a college class). The treatment itself cost me nothing, but more important is that just 30 days after I started my therapy, I regained control over my life and I no longer had headaches.

But what is aroma-conditioning? What did I learn about the psychology of learning that made me think of aroma-conditioning? Who was the man with a white beard who inspired me? Migraine can't be cured (most people who claim they can cure migraine are using the word *cure* as a sales pitch). But I did get rid of migraine headaches. The rest of this book explains how I manage to ward off headaches and how you can too. I'll show you how the concepts of learning from psychology relate to migraine. Migraine is a biological, not a psychological illness—why is it possible to treat it with methods from psychology? The book gives answers to these and other questions.

The Chapters

Chapter I shows the basic differences between common types of headaches. Because aroma-conditioning treats migraine, it's important to make a distinction between migraine and other headache symptoms.

Chapter II briefly examines what migraine is and how it is usually treated. To understand aroma-conditioning, you need to understand the migraine attack phases and the difference between pain-relieving (abortive) and preventive medications and treatments for migraines.

Chapter III, designed as an assessment phase for my psychological experiment, shows how aromatherapy relates to my successful treatment with aroma-conditioning.

Chapter IV reveals step by step how I came to live without migraine headaches, using aroma-conditioning therapy. It also presents evidence for aroma-conditioning as a therapy.

Chapter V describes the critical steps and elements of aroma-conditioning as a therapy for migraines.

Chapter VI helps you gain a clear understanding of classical conditioning as a form of learning, which is the key to aroma-conditioning. It also brings up the psychological perspective that influenced my development of aroma-conditioning as a migraine therapy.

Chapter VII demonstrates how classical conditioning can account for drug effects; it also explains the role of expectations and classical conditioning in the placebo effect phenomenon.

Chapter VIII shows how I approached my new idea for aroma-conditioning therapy—as a scientific experiment in behavioral psychology.

Appendix A contains two effective relaxation techniques for migraine headaches that I learned and tested on myself. The breathing technique can be combined with aroma-conditioning for a greater effect.

CHAPTER I

MIGRAINES AND OTHER HEADACHES

Because aroma-conditioning treats migraines, it is important to learn more about headaches and how other types of headaches are different from migraine.

The pain of headaches doesn't develop in the brain; the brain itself is not sensitive to pain. Instead, headaches begin in the areas surrounding the brain—tissues covering the brain, and blood vessels and muscles around the face, neck, and scalp. Headaches fall into two main categories: primary and secondary.

Secondary headaches are symptoms of another health problem. Some of them are signs of a minor problem such as a cold or flu; others are caused by a serious condition—neck and head injuries, stroke, or sinus infection. High blood pressure and some medications may also trigger headaches.

Primary Headaches

Primary headaches account for about 95% of all headaches and are not caused by another medical condition. Instead, they originate from factors such as stress, hormonal imbalances, or fatigue. Primary headaches are tension-type headaches and neurovascular headaches (migraine and cluster headaches).

Headaches are also categorized as episodic or chronic. Episodic headaches are headaches you have once in a while. If you have headaches more than 15 days each month, you have chronic headaches. Most chronic headaches are primary, either tension-type or migraine headaches.

Tension-Type Headaches

Tension-type headaches are the most common primary headaches and the most common headaches of all (about 90%). Headache specialists once thought that tension and spasms in the muscles in the neck, face, and scalp were the main cause for tension-type headaches. Today they believe that biochemical abnormalities may also cause tension-type headaches. Depression, anxiety, stress, eyestrain, and poor posture can lead to tension-type headaches.

People with tension-type headaches describe the pain as steady and tightening, felt around the neck, back of the head, or the forehead. The pain may last from 30 minutes to hours and days. Frequency varies.

Neurovascular Headaches

Neurovascular headaches, migraines (see Chapter III, "Migraine: More than a Headache.") and cluster headaches, are common primary headaches. They used to be known as vascular disorders—blood vessels constrict and reduce blood flow to the brain and then dilate and the dilation causes the pain. The newer theory is that biochemical imbalances in the brain cause the change in the blood flow.

The symptoms of cluster headaches are easy to distinguish from those of migraine. The pain, usually more intense than that of migraine, is piercing, drill-like and felt in or around one of the eyes. The painful eye may become red and tear up and the nostril on the painful side can become runny. Cluster headaches occur suddenly and last from 30 to 90 minutes. A person suffering from cluster headaches can have several episodes per day for weeks or months.

Mixed Headaches

People with migraine may experience tension-type headaches, and people who have chronic tension-type headaches may start having migraine symptoms like pre-headache or sensitivity to light and sound during an attack. Headaches that have characteristics of both migraine and tension-type headaches are known as mixed headaches. They are sometimes classified as a third type of migraine.

Migraines can cause tension-type headaches. Having a chronic migraine may lead to muscle tension, and the tension may cause tension-type headaches. Because headaches can easily mutate from one type to another, resulting in mix symptoms—diagnosis can be a challenge.

Chronic Daily Headaches

Chronic daily headaches are headaches that appear every day or almost every day. They usually develop from chronic migraine or tension-type headaches. People with migraine who have daily headaches often start to feel the steady, dull pain that is typical of tension-type headaches. Aura symptoms (visual disturbances felt by some people with migraines) may also become milder over time. At the same time, people with tension-type headaches may begin to experience nausea, vomiting and sharp throbbing pain—all characteristic of migraine.

> **Distinguishing Tension-Type Headaches from Migraine Headaches**
>
> Tension-type headaches are sometimes difficult to distinguish from migraine. One important difference between the two is that tension-type headaches can be much more frequent than migraine—chronic tension-type headaches can occur almost every day, while typical chronic migraine headaches occur 2-3 times a month. Chronic migraine headaches usually last longer—4 hours or more; chronic tension-type headaches often last 30 minutes. The pain of migraine is usually throbbing; the pain of tension-type headache is steady. Vomiting, nausea, and sensitivity to light, sound, and motion are common symptoms for migraine, but they do not usually accompany tension-type headaches.

About half the cases of chronic daily headaches are caused by overusing over-the-counter or prescription painkillers. Daily headaches that result from medication overuse are called rebound headaches.

Rebound headaches develop gradually. It may take years until they transform into chronic daily headaches. The pain of rebound daily headaches is often less intense, but people who have them experience severe headaches more frequently. The best way to treat rebound headaches is to stop all medications at once, but only under a doctor's care. If your daily headaches are actually caused by the medication, you will improve quickly.

Diagnosing Your Headaches

To diagnose your headaches, a doctor will first consider your medical history and headache symptoms. If the pattern of symptoms is a hallmark of a particular type of headaches, this may be enough to confirm a diagnosis. To rule out other, dangerous causes of headaches that resemble primary headaches, your doctor may recommend diagnostic tests—blood tests, CT or MRI scans.

CHAPTER II

MIGRAINE: MORE THAN
A HEADACHE

"As a child, I used to cry when I woke up with a severe migraine head-ache. I felt guilty every time I deprived my parents of their sleep and kept them up late while they tried soothing me. When I learned more about gender roles, I stopped crying and went on to suffer in silence."

What Does a Migraine Feel Like?

Imagine today is one of those beautiful summer days and you're about to start your family vacation. You're excited and full of happy thoughts and feelings. As you prepare for the trip, you feel a slight tingling sensation inside your head. You feel it but you are not yet aware of it because you're busy.

You begin to yawn and feel sleepy, your eyes are watery, and your vision is a little blurred. The tingling sensation has grown to a sharp pulsing feeling on the left side of your head. You know a headache is coming and you get a little frustrated. Five minutes later, the pulsing turns to pain and the pain becomes stronger and sharper. The bright sun of the beautiful summer day becomes a terrible nuisance—it intensifies the pain as does any sound. You go to the darkest room to lie down and you cover your eyes with a blanket. You can't talk and you can't move because any activity makes things worse.

Now imagine a blacksmith hammering out the lower back side of your head and then he switches with a jackhammer operator for an hour or two. After the hammering and jackhammering, if you haven't fallen asleep, you have a pulsing feeling inside your head—sharp pain that alternates with no pain; then two times no pain, sharp pain, until it disappears.

You feel physically exhausted, as if *you* have been a jackhammer operator, working all day fixing roads. You're late for the trip—you were supposed to start driving three hours ago. But you feel a bit lucky: What if I had this bad headache yesterday at work?

Migraines Are Inherited

Most people associate the words *migraine* and *migraines* with headaches. But as my example of what migraines feel like, there's a lot more about migraines than that. Migraines are an illness caused by a biochemical abnormality in the brain. A person born with this abnormality is very sensitive to certain types of stimuli called migraine triggers.

A migraine trigger starts a migraine attack, or migraine episode. The trigger causes a biochemical reaction that starts a series of sensations. Anything in a person's lifestyle or environment can become a migraine trigger—stress, excitement, sunlight, bright light, and certain foods and drinks. Sometimes a combination of stimuli can be a trigger, which can make migraine triggers difficult to recognize.

Migraine Symptoms and Phases (Migraine Attack)

A person with migraines, even one who suffers from the most acute migraine symptoms, is and looks normal most of the time. But during a migraine attack (an instance of migraine), a set of changes occur throughout that person's body. The migraine I described in the beginning of this chapter is my typical migraine, but for other people symptoms like nausea and vomiting are also a part of their migraines.

If you ask two people who have migraines to describe what they feel during an episode, you will notice a similar pattern. At first, symptoms build up to a severe pain and then they diminish. Symptoms of a migraine attack may last 30 minutes, several hours, or even days. Migraine specialists refer to this pattern as the migraine phases: preheadache, aura, headache, and postheadache. Not all patients, however, experience the four phases of migraine.

Preheadache (Prodrome)

Preheadache is a set of symptoms that may precede a migraine attack. They usually begin a couple of minutes or several hours before the headache phase. Mood changes, sensitivity to light and sound, yawning, dizziness, neck stiffness, and mood changes are examples of preheadache symptoms.

Aura

Some people may also experience sensory disturbances minutes before the migraine pain starts. Visual effects like sparkling or flashing zigzags, swirls, or white spots, and blurred vision are common aura symptoms. Some migraine patients may, on occasion, experience aura without pain and preheadache.

Migraines are often classified as migraine with aura (common migraine) or migraine without aura (classic migraine), and a person with migraine may experience both at different times. Most people have migraines without aura.

Headache

Migraine headaches usually occur on one side of the head, most often around the temples, which is the reason for the name of the illness; the word migraine originates from the Greek word *hemikrania* (half of the head). Sometimes the headache might spread through the entire head and parts of the body. People describe the pain as pulsating or throbbing.

The headache is the most severe symptom of migraine, but in addition to the pain at this stage, many migraine patients have to deal with vomiting and nausea. During the headache phase, light, sound, and motion worsen the pain. The headache phase may last from four to several hours and can start without preheadache or an aura, especially at night during sleep.

Postheadache (Postdrome)

After the headache, some people with migraines might experience physical and mental exhaustion. These symptoms are known as postheadache phase or postdrome.

Managing Migraine Headaches

Migraine headaches are a chronic condition that can't be cured. No known cure for migraines exists. But like other chronic disorders, migraines can be managed. Migraine management involves controlling the symptoms, reducing the number of migraines and their intensity, and avoiding migraine triggers.

Migraines are treated with two basic approaches—symptom-relieving (abortive) and preventive. Symptom-relieving drugs are usually taken at fist signs of a migraine attack to stop a headache from developing. The goal of preventive treatment for migraines is to reduce the frequency and intensity of migraines.

Treating Migraines with Symptom-Relieving (Abortive) Drugs

Over-the-Counter Medications (Painkillers)

Even though migraines are a leading cause for disability, more than a half of the people with migraines rely on over-the-counter medications for relief. Unfortunately, these medications can only help those who have less severe and less frequent migraine headaches. Why then are OTC drugs so popular? Easy access, low cost, and advertising are some possible reasons, but many people with migraines have too little knowledge of their condition. Remember that overusing OTC drugs leads to chronic daily headaches. (See Chapter II, "Migraines and Other Headaches.")

Aspirin, acetaminophen (Tylenol), ibuprofen (Advil Migraine) are the three most common OTC drugs. Clinical studies have shown that the three are equally effective in preventing or relieving mild migraine headaches.

Prescription Drugs

Ergots are a family of abortive drugs for migraines. They are the oldest prescription drugs for treating migraines and have been in use since the 1920's. Ergots contract blood vessels, and stimulate the production of serotonin in the brain. The most common ergot is ergotamine (Cafergot), which is often mixed with caffeine for a greater effect. Ergotamine can relief pain and sometimes reduce the number of migraine headaches. This drug must be used with caution: overusing ergotamine can cause serious health problems, including prolonged spasms of the arteries or severe daily headaches.

Many people with migraines find a relief in a family of drugs called **triptans**. Like ergots, triptans also constrict blood vessels. These drugs are safer than ergots and they come in pills, nasal sprays, or injections. In the United States, some common drugs from this family are sumatriptan (Imitrex), naratriptan (Amerge), frovatriptan (Frova), rizatriptan (Maxalt), almotriptan (Axert), and zolmitriptan (Zomig).

Treating Migraines with Preventive Drugs

A preventive therapy must be considered for people who have frequent migraine headaches, or for those who use painkillers too often. Most preventive drugs should be taken daily. Preventive drugs become less effective with time. Once a medication becomes ineffective, the patient must switch to a different drug. Most of these medications were not originally intended for migraines.

Currently there are four preventive drugs approved by FDA: the **beta-blockers:** propranolol (Inderal), timolol (Blocadren), and the **anticonvulsants**: divalproex sodium (Depakote) and topiramate (Topamax).

Non-Drug Treatments for Migraines

Non-drug treatments for migraines can also be classified as symptom-relieving and preventive. Avoiding triggers, for example, is a preventive therapy, and relaxation techniques are symptom-relieving. Relaxation techniques can also be preventive; if you prevent enough migraine headaches using a relaxation technique, your migraine headaches may become less frequent—just what a preventive therapy is supposed to do. Effective and easy to learn self-help relaxation techniques are Progressive Muscle Relaxation and Slowing Down Respiration. (See Appendix).

Experts say that avoiding migraine triggers and making lifestyle changes can reduce the severity and frequency of migraines. Migraine triggers are not easy to identify and are different for every patient. To identify migraine triggers, experts recommend keeping a headache diary to identify patterns and migraine triggers.

Psychology and Migraines

Why treat physiological illness like migraine with psychology? Let's answer this question using the learning perspective in psychology. Learning can produce not only psychological but physiological responses in humans. Take for example social phobia—an excessive fear of social situations. Social phobia makes people anxious and anxiety causes physical changes like increased heart rate, perspiration, and muscle tightness.

A person with migraines whose main trigger is anxiety produced by social phobia can go through counterconditioning with the help of a psychotherapist. And as the phobia disappears in the treatment process, anxiety and physical changes produced by it will go too. And so will the migraine headaches.

With the help of trained psychologists, some people with migraines find relief in behavior therapies like biofeedback, relaxation training, stress-management training, or hypnotherapy, usually in combination with a drug therapy. These therapies can be as helpful as pharmacological therapies but they can cost more and many people with migraine do not have access to them.

Aroma-conditioning, on the other hand, is a behavior therapy that can be used without the help of a trained psychologist and costs nothing, compared to other behavior therapies.

Important Words

Understanding these words is important for understanding migraine and the main idea of this book.

migraine: the illness that causes migraine headaches and other symptoms like nausea and sensitivity to light and sound

a migraine (migraines) / a migraine headache (migraine headaches): a headache (headaches) caused by the illness migraine

preheadache (prodrome): symptoms like sensitivity to light and sound that usually precede a migraine headache

migraine attack: an instance of migraine, a process during which you may experience a number of symptoms including a headache; a migraine attack can consist of preheadache symptoms like sensitivity to light and sound

symptom-relieving (abortive) drugs for migraine: a drug for stopping the process of a migraine attack; ideally a symptom-relieving drug should prevent the headache phase of a migraine attack when taken at the first preheadache signs

migraine trigger: anything that could start a migraine attack; certain foods, stress and anxiety, bright light, or a combination of things can be migraine triggers

CHAPTER III

MIGRAINES, DRUGS, AND AROMATHERAPY

Doing Science with a Ringing Bell

After noticing the curious behavior of the dog, the man with a white beard quickly abandoned his research on digestion and devised the most famous experiment in psychology. He wanted to see if he could teach a dog to salivate on ringing of a bell, since the dog seemed to have learned to salivate on hearing his footsteps without training. So, as part of the experiment, the man sounded a bell every time before he gave food to the dog. Eventually, the dog salivated once it heard the ringing. The dog learned to respond to something—the sound of a bell—the same way it responded, as a natural instinct, to seeing the food; in other words, the dog learned to associate the sound of a bell with food.

What was the significance of this? The man with a white beard discovered, by chance, the most basic way humans and other organisms learn; a way of learning that helps organisms survive in and adapt to the world. This type of learning is now known as classical conditioning. Before discussing classical conditioning further, let's consider what learning is.

For most people, learning is the act of gaining knowledge or skill, usually by study or instruction. For psychologists, learning has a broader meaning—a dog shaking hands, a child playing a musical instrument, or a dolphin leaping into the air on the signal of a trainer are all examples of behavior acquired through learning, which can happen almost everywhere, to almost every living organism at any stage of its life.

This means that humans and other living things use similar methods to learn from experience. Any experience can lead to learning. And we know that learning takes place when someone or something changes their usual behavior.

Before Conditioning

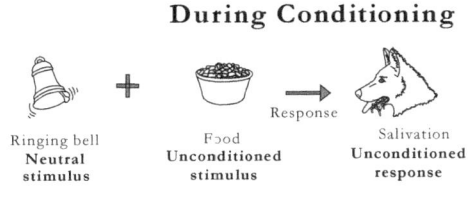

Ringing bell
Neutral stimulus

No salivation
Neutral response

and

Food
Unconditioned stimulus

Salivation
Unconditioned response

Before conditioning, the ringing bell is a neutral stimulus. The dog hears the bell but doesn't salivate or respond in any way. Food is unconditioned stimulus. When the dog sees the food, it salivates.

During Conditioning

Ringing bell
Neutral stimulus

Food
Unconditioned stimulus

Salivation
Unconditioned response

During conditioning the ringing bell (the neutral stimulus) is frequently sounded before the food (the unconditioned stimulus) is presented. The dog salivates.

After Conditioning

Ringing bell
Conditioned stimulus

Salivation
Conditioned response

After conditioning, the ringing bell alone makes the dog salivate. At this stage, the ringing of a bell is the conditioned stimulus and the salivation is the conditioned response.

Figure 1
Classical Conditioning

In the ringing-bell experiment (Figure 1), the dog did change its usual behavior—it became apt to drooling whenever it heard a ringing bell. We can also say that the dog was classically-conditioned. What are the main elements of this type of learning?

The dog food is called the **unconditioned stimulus**—the dog's natural response to food was salivation. The drooling, a natural reflex, produced by the unconditioned stimulus is called the **unconditioned response**. Before the experiment, the ringing bell was a **neutral stimulus** because the dog did not react to it in any way. After the experiment, however, the ringing bell became a **conditioned stimulus**—because at that point the dog was apt to salivate when it heard the bell. The response (salivation) to a conditioned stimulus is called a **conditioned response**. To learn more about the ringing bell theory and how to make the most of it to get rid of migraines, go to Chapter VI, "The Man with a White Beard."

But more important is that drug effects can be classically conditioned. (See Chapter VII, "Drug Effects, the Ringing Bell Theory, and the Mighty Placebo.") The man with a white beard was the first who proposed that the curing effects of a drug could be transferred to something harmless, like a sense of smell or taste. Say you successfully pair a neutral stimulus like a sense of smell with a drug used for treating a physiological illness; the harmless smell will become the instrument of the treatment. Transferring the curing effects of a powerful medicine for migraines, using the ringing bell theory, was the idea I had while lying in bed helpless.

Trapped by Migraines

Helplessness and pain in the dark bring back some of my earliest childhood memories and are things I associate with the word *migraines*. I've had migraine headaches since I was three years old. Concerned about my health, my parents dragged me across Bulgaria to see various headache specialists. No one diagnosed my headaches as migraines until I was seven.

After my parents learned that my headaches were actually migraines and not other serious condition, they got some relief. My mother started a migraine diary for me and she recorded everything about the days I had migraine headaches. She still keeps this diary, plus all the paperwork related to my childhood migraines, including physical examinations, EEG results, drug prescriptions, etc.

My migraine symptoms changed over time. Many years ago, I felt the sharp pain above my left eye. But my headache have gradually spread to include the left back side of my head. The pain started to feel steady and dull, more like the tension-type headaches. When in pain, I also started to feel tightness in the left part of the neck and shoulder. My shoulder started to grow so stiff during migraine headaches, that I once asked a 300-pound guy to hit my shoulder repeatedly, using all his strength. Believe it or not, I felt relief after each and every blow of his fist.

The stiffness appeared at the same time as my headaches became more frequent. The change in my migraine symptoms has been very gradual, and over a period of about 15 years.

Until I was eighteen, I had migraine headaches about once a month. After that, I started having headaches once or two times a week. In the last five years before my experiment, things had gotten even worse. I had started to have chronic daily headaches lasting from about 30 minutes to one or two hours.

My Migraines Just before Aroma-Conditioning

At the time of my experiment with aroma-conditioning I had 4-5 headaches a week. My headaches lasted from 30 minutes to one or two hours. My headaches usually developed in the afternoon, but it wasn't uncommon to start my day with a headache. I awoke with a sharp throbbing headache once or twice a month.

Most of my migraine headaches started with pre-headache symptoms. At first, my vision blurred and my eyes became watery. This was where people who knew me said, "Are you going to have a headache?" At the same time, I started to feel sleepy, had a tingling sensation inside my head. Then light and sound started to irritate me. I felt dizzy. Just before the headache, I felt stiffness on the left side of my neck.

During my headache phase, the pain was just above my left eye and on the lower back left side of my head. Sometimes my whole head was in pain, and rarely did it switch to the area above my right eye. I remember having preheadaches without actual headache only a couple of times. Preheadaches without migraines are more common among other people with migraine headaches. During most of my migraine headaches I needed bed rest in a dark and quiet place.

Most of my migraine headaches resulted in severe pain. Here is the frequency pain levels I had during my migraine headaches just before my experiment with aroma-conditioning:

No pain   0%

Mild pain   2%

Moderate pain   5%

Severe pain   80%

Excruciating pain 13%

When in severe or excruciating pain, I had to keep my eyes shut and covered, because the slightest light increased the pain. Sound and movement also increased the pain. After the headache phase, I felt physically and mentally exhausted.

I had several headache triggers. One was staying near bright light too long or in front of a computer screen. But the most common were emotion and stress. People close to me noticed that if I got worried, angry, or enthusiastic, I was apt to get a headache. When my wife and I were about to go on vacation, she'd say, "Don't get too excited, you'll get a headache." My mother said that as a child, if I played an exciting game with other children, I would get a headache and wake everyone up at night. Emotions are a great part of my personality.

At the time of my experiment, I smoked on average 20 cigarettes a day. Nicotine was a possible migraine trigger. I couldn't prove it though, because I couldn't see a pattern. I am also nearsighted and have a strong prescription. Since I started wearing contact lenses before high-school, my nearsightedness has never bothered me. I often find myself seeing better than people with healthier eyes. There could be a relationship between my migraine headaches and my nearsightedness, but I had no means of finding out.

At the time of my experiment with migraine treatment I was 29. I had just moved to the United States in 2003, as an international student, and got married in 2004. I was still a student when I started my therapy.

Another of my important characteristics, as a migraine patient, is my gender as an adult man. More adult women have migraines than men, so women appear to be more representative of people with migraines in an experiment involving migraines. But this is not necessarily the case. A larger number of women migraine sufferers can be explained by the greater number of hormonal events a woman experiences: menstrual cycles, pregnancy, and menopause. These events contribute to chemical imbalances in the body and are potential triggers for any woman born with the chemical abnormality that causes migraines. A woman's change of body chemistry caused by pregnancy is similar to the change of my body chemistry when I'm emotional—they are both potential migraine triggers. Triggers start migraine episodes.

Drug Effects I Wanted to Transfer with the Ringing Bell Theory

I relied on over-the-counter medications for relief—paracetamol, ibuprofen, aspirin or any similar analgesic. I have used Advil and Exedrin in the United States, and some European brands. I don't know how and if these analgesics worked, but I took pills in search for headache relief.

I last visited a migraine specialist six years ago in Bulgaria. It was several months before I moved to the states. The doctor prescribed Coffergamine, a prescription drug equivalent to the pain-reliever for migraines Cafergot. Coffergamine is a mix of ergotamine and caffeine. Most medications that contain ergotamine have caffeine for a greater effect. Ergotamine is prescribed for acute migraines and works by affecting the serotonin, dopamine, and adrenaline neurotransmitters. It also constricts blood vessels, which is how it reduces inflammation and pain. I had no side effects from using ergotamine.

Side Effects of Ergotamine

Taking ergotamine more than twice a week may lead to rebound headaches. On rare occasions, it is known to cause permanent spasms of the blood vessels, which can lead to serious health problems. Though this happens rarely, ergotamine must be used with caution because of the serious complications associated with a permanent spasm of blood vessels—heart problems or gangrene, the symptoms of which can be chest pain or paleness of fingers and toes.

Other symptoms from excessive use of ergotamine can be muscle pain, chest pain, leg pain when walking, coldness, abnormally pale fingers and toes, numbness, fluid retention, weakness, high blood pressure, nausea, vomiting, and vertigo. Ergotamine can also cause psychological dependence and if discontinued it can cause severe headaches or other withdrawal problems.

I tried the ergotamine and caffeine drug several times after my doctor prescribed it. But I don't remember it having any effect. I might not have taken it in time. Pain-relieving drugs like ergotamine are effective when taken right after the first preheadache symptoms. After I moved to the States my headaches worsened. So I was forced to become active in managing my migraine headaches. But I wanted to avoid going back to a migraine specialist, so I tried the ergotamine pills again.

I remember vividly the first two occasions I took ergotamine. It had been years since I felt preheadache symptoms without later having a migraine headache. With the pills, I was able to prevent 90% of my migraine headaches. I had about 40 migraine attacks in two months. If I took a pill right after my first preheadache symptoms, I didn't have a headache. But because of the many side effects, you can't take ergotamine every day. I became concerned and wondered how long can I keep taking this medicine. With the headaches no other health risk was involved. In the end, I decided to stop using the medicine.

Because I quit taking the ergotamine drug, my next preheadache developed into a full-blown migraine headache. Soon I was back to my cycle of daily headaches.

I spent two weeks in agony, until my idea for migraine therapy struck me. I wanted to see if the effects of ergotamine could be transferred to something safe, using classical conditioning.

How Did I Choose Peppermint Oil for Aroma-Conditioning?

After the man with a white beard, another researcher paired sweetened water with a powerful medication that suppressed the immune system of a lab animal. After a number of pairings, the sweetened water alone suppressed the immune system. For people suffering from autoimmune disorders, suppressing the immune system is the desired effect of treatment. (See Chapter VII, "Drug Effects, the Ringing Bell Theory, and the Mighty Placebo.")

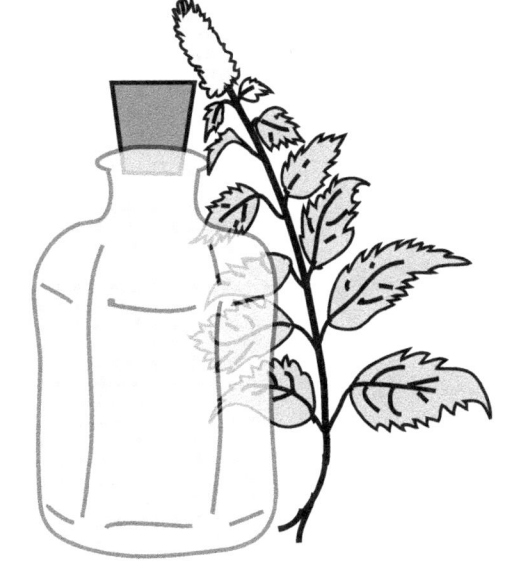

Like the researcher who succeeded using sweetened water to suppress the immune system, I wanted to see if peppermint oil could be used to suppress migraines, after pairing it with a medicine. But why peppermint oil? I couldn't use just any taste or smell. Something part of my daily diet would not work. Take coffee, for example. I drank coffee every day but didn't have migraine headaches every day. On most occasions I would drink coffee without needing to prevent migraine headaches, which would have made classical conditioning impossible. To achieve a conditioned response, the medicine and the sense of smell must always appear together. (See Chapter VI, "The Man with a White Beard.")

33

The best smell or taste for my medical experiment was something that I liked, that made me feel well by itself. I liked a lot the smell and taste of peppermint oil. Inhaling the aroma of peppermint oil (a couple of drops near my nose and on my forehead) made me feel relaxed. It's also important that although the mint aroma made me feel better during migraine headaches before I started my treatment with classical conditioning, mint never prevented my headaches.

The pleasant effects of peppermint are from personal experience. Since I was 5-years-old, every time I had a migraine headache, my mother soothed me by rubbing peppermint oil on my forehead. Over time, I associated the smell of mint with this experience. The experience of my mother rubbing peppermint oil on my forehead is an example of classical conditioning. The gentle care of my mother paired with the smell of peppermint, and eventually the smell of mint became a conditioned stimulus for a pleasant emotional response.

The Ringing Bell Theory and Peppermint

Why did my mother treat me with mint oil? As a traditional medicine enthusiast, she knew about the analgesic qualities of the plant. Peppermint oil, a very popular aromatherapy product, has been known to relive headaches for many years. In fact, it can relieve various kinds of pain. When applied to the skin, peppermint oil has a cooling effect and produces local anesthesia and muscle relaxation, which relieves pain. Inhaling peppermint oil can soothe the respiratory system producing relaxation, which also contributes to pain relief.

Before my experiment, peppermint oil alone had never prevented the headache phase of my migraine attacks, although it was one of my favorite pain relievers. When I applied peppermint oil directly where my head hurt (diluting it with water, dropping a few drops on a wet towel and use as a compress) I felt a moderate and pleasant loss of sensation and my muscles relaxed, which reduced the pain. The oil also helped me breathe easier, opening my airways. This, and my fondness for the aroma, made me feel relaxed overall.

Peppermint

Peppermint (*Mentha Piperita*) is a well-known perennial herb, a natural hybrid of spearmint and water mint. Because of its many uses in the food industry, cosmetics, and medicine—peppermint is cultivated throughout the world. The specific strong taste and aroma of peppermint come from the volatile oils contained it its leaves and stems. Both in Europe and America peppermint oil is obtained from the fresh, above-ground parts of the plant. The main component of the oil is Menthol.

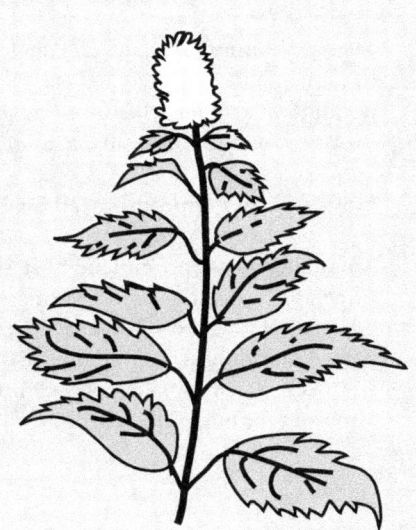

The plant's oils are known to have muscle-relaxing, analgesic, and even antibacterial qualities. Besides headaches, peppermint is used to treat stomach ailments, menstrual cramps, skin irritation, colds, flu, nausea, anxiety, and daytime sleepiness. According to the International Journal of Toxicology (2001, p. 65), peppermint oil can improve cognitive performance.

A study by researchers at the University of Northumbria in England provided further evidence of how peppermint aroma impacts brain activity and mood. Of the 144 volunteers in the study, those who sniffed the aroma of peppermint improved their memory and alertness.

Scientific Research on Peppermint as Migraine Remedy

There's scientific evidence confirming that peppermint can help relieve headaches; German researchers Gobel, Schmidt, and Soyka (1994) at Neurological Clinic of the University of Kiel devised a study and concluded that essential plant oils of peppermint are very effective for headache management (as cited in McCaleb, 1995).

The Peppermint Oil Used in My Experiment

The peppermint oil I used was made according to the European standards by Bulgarian company Chemax Pharma. I brought three bottles of peppermint oil with me when I moved to the States. I used this peppermint oil because it was readily available to me.

How To Use Peppermint Oil for Headaches

Aromatherapists recommend that peppermint oil be diluted with water when applied on the skin. For migraine, you can add a few drops of mint oil on a cold, wet towel and apply it to your forehead or wherever you feel pain. You can also use the diluted oil to massage your forehead, temples, and neck. When inhaled, peppermint oil can relieve nausea—a common symptom for migraine patients.

Aromatherapy

Aromatherapy is a type of alternative medicine that uses essential plant oils believed to have psychological and physical healing properties. Essential oils are extracted from leaves, roots, stems or other plant parts. Usually essential oils are

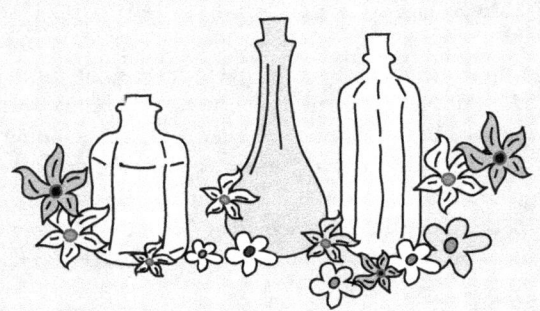

diluted with vegetable oils, also known as carrier oils. Essential oils can be applied to the skin or inhaled. Fragrances or perfume oils are synthetic oils that are different than essential oils used in aromatherapy.

How Does It Work?

The smell of essential oils directly affects the limbic system, the part of the brain that controls emotions. The smell of essential oils enters the limbic system through the olfactory system, the system responsible for our sense of smell. And because pleasant smells stimulate emotional responses of pleasure, they can also aid relaxation and reduce stress. As pleasant smells make you feel good and relaxed, you will be less likely to succumb to stress-related disorders and physiological illnesses. If you have migraine and your main triggers are stress and anxiety, it makes sense to try aromatherapy.

Purpose

Since ancient times, essential oils have been used for healing wounds, strengthening the immune system, improving memory, or relieving stress. They are also used as a holistic therapy. These properties of essential oils haven't been adequately supported by academic research. Nevertheless, many physicians consider aromatherapy as a useful complementary treatment for many psychological disorders like anxiety, depression, and insomnia. Many people find relief for ailments and pains using aromatherapy without the side effects of prescription drugs.

How to Use

Often used externally in massages, essential oils can also be applied to the skin in the form of compresses. Essential oils can be inhaled directly, sprayed in the room, or inhaled with steam. Some oils are used in hand or foot baths to treat sore muscles, arthritis, or skin conditions. Many people take full body baths for beauty and relaxation. Home aromatherapy products are available on the market—from essential oils for bath or massage, to oils you can burn in a candle or spray in the room.

Safety

The United States does not regulate the use of the word aromatherapy on product labels or the production of essential oils. So, it is a good practice to purchase essential oils from reliable sources and check the labels of products for ingredients and for expiration dates. Synthetic ingredients and substitutions are not the same as essential oils derived from plants—they don't have the healing properties of essential oils. Natural essential oils are more expensive to manufacture and are often substituted with synthetics. Because essential oils and their carrier oils deteriorate quickly, aromatherapists recommend the use of fresh essential oils.

What to Expect

Generally, aromatherapy is considered safe when used externally on the skin or inhaled. Most people who use aromatherapy get a feeling of emotional and physical relaxation. Some people may develop allergies or skin irritation.

CHAPTER IV

AROMA-CONDITIONING
IN ACTION

Feel, Pill, Inhale

The day after I had the idea for treating migraines, I thought as soon as I felt a migraine headache coming, I would swallow a pill, inhale the peppermint oil directly from the bottle, apply a drop or two of the oil directly under my nose and breathe deeply. Deep breaths would make my entire body aware of the peppermint as an unconditioned stimulus. I though that the stimulus, peppermint oil, must be felt clearly by both my skin and lungs; according to classical conditioning theory, the stronger the stimulus, the stronger the conditioning effect.

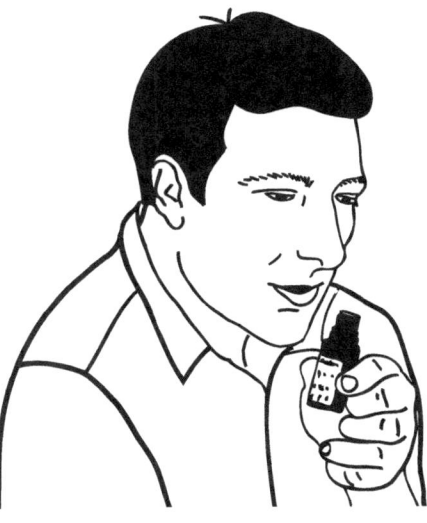

So I went on and prepared. I took out one peppermint bottle from the fridge and examined it to make sure there was enough liquid to last me for several migraines. I made sure I had enough ergotamine pills. I bundled together the bottle of oil and the blister packs of ergotamine pills and from then on, these became my classical conditioning kit or, even better, my aroma-conditioning kit. They were always going to be in my pocket, until I no longer relied on the pills, that is if the classical conditioning worked.

A day later I felt a migraine headache coming. I was working. I swallowed an ergotamine pill, inhaled the peppermint oil from the bottle, applied the oil under my nose, breathed in and out deeply. I felt the freshness of the menthol vapor. This lasted two minutes, and I went back to work. I felt the usual preheadache sensations like the stiffness in my neck and the dizziness and I started yawning. Those symptoms, however, didn't turn into a headache. I expected that. It was the ergotamine, which had prevented my headache phase during the previous two months.

I kept having migraine attacks 4-5 times a week as usual, and I stuck to my plan meticulously. I never forgot to bring my aroma-conditioning kit. As soon as I felt sick, I would first take the pill, with a glass of water, and then inhale. I never missed the peppermint oil and never forgot to take the medication right upon the first preheadache sings of every migraine attack. Two weeks later, it became a routine—preheadache, pill, inhalation of peppermint oil.

Which Should Come First—Aroma or Medication?

According to classical conditioning theorists, the unconditioned stimulus should come first in order for conditioning to be effective. I forgot this and made a habit of inhaling the peppermint oil first.

Not that researchers say it's impossible to produce conditioning in the way I did it, but it goes a little against the cognitive theory of classical conditioning. According to classical conditioning theory, the unconditioned stimulus should accurately predict the appearance of the conditioned stimulus and prepare the organism for an important biological event.

Using terms from behavioral psychology, the period of my initial pairing was the response acquisition phase of classical conditioning. At first, the inhalation of peppermint oil was a neutral stimulus—although it improved my general sense of well-being, it had nothing to do with preventing the headache phase of my migraines. The drug did. The preventing of my headache phases was the unconditioned response naturally caused by the medicine. The unconditioned stimulus was the medicine, and each paring of medicine and peppermint oil was what research psychologists call a trial. (See Chapter "The Man with a White Beard.")

> **How Many Times I Paired Aroma with Drug**
>
> I did not count the number of times I paired the medicine with the inhalation. But I guess it might have been between 16-20 time, according to the number of migraine attacks I had per month.

The Sicker the Better?

I had fulfilled the classical conditioning requirements. I always presented the neutral stimulus, the peppermint oil, within seconds of the unconditioned stimulus, the medicine. I never let one stimulus appear without the other, i.e. use the medicine without inhaling the peppermint oil or the reverse. I was careful to take the medicine on time, so that it actually prevented the headache phases of my migraine attacks when I paired it with the peppermint oil. Otherwise, I would have no response to classically condition.

I fulfilled two more important requirements—frequent and enough pairings, which involved some sort of scientific irony. According to the classical conditioning theory, the more frequently you pair the neutral and unconditioned stimulus, the stronger the learning. It's the same with the number of pairings—the more, the stronger. And during the first month of my aroma-conditioning, I had migraine attacks almost every day of the week, 4-5 times, which is a very unpleasant situation. But that was a perfect opportunity for frequent and numerous pairings or, as psychologists call them, trials.

What does this mean? The sicker you are with headaches, the likelier it is to transfer the effects of a medicine with classical conditioning, getting rid of the medicine and becoming healthier. That's the scientific irony.

My First Headache Prevented with Aroma-Conditioning

In the first month, none of my migraine attacks developed into a headache, thanks to the medicine. I didn't know how long I had to keep pairing the medicine with the peppermint oil. I even put off stopping the pills, afraid the headaches would make my life miserable again. One day, I rushed to work and only remembered to take the bottle of oil on my way out the door. Within hours, I felt dizzy and stiff and about to have a headache and I found my aroma-conditioning kit was incomplete. I had finished the pills.

The restaurant was packed. A long line of customers were outside, waiting to be seated by me. The waiters were unable to take care of more tables, so I had to juggle the role of a host and waiter. With the pre-headache I was having, I had no time for my other set of roles—as a researcher and patient. I quickly decided to inhale the peppermint oil. I saw this as an opportunity to see if my efforts were worthy of the man with a white beard.

For the first time, I used the peppermint oil without the medicine. I popped open the bottle of peppermint oil and breathed in the fresh menthol smell. I applied a couple of drops under my nose with my index finger, and breathed in and out deeply several times. My preheadache symptoms lasted 5-10 minutes, but the headache never came. I though it was some kind of coincidence. Was this the first time I managed to prevent a headache using aroma-conditioning?

How Aroma-Conditioning Improved My Migraine Symptoms

I decided it must have been the conditioning. Previously without the medicine, each of my preheadaches resulted in a headache. I remember only a couple of occasions throughout my life when I had preheadache symptoms that did not turn into a migraine headache.

The following day, I had another migraine attack. I inhaled the peppermint oil, breathing in and out deeply. In five minutes I felt as good as new. Since then, with aroma-conditioning, I prevented each headache whenever I had a migraine attack, for about 12 months. That is, not a minute of migraine headaches.

In the first three months of that period, I had migraine attacks as frequently as before, 4-5 per week. But none turned into a headache. Because I had suffered from horrible pain every day, I had started to expect to suffer every day. I felt anxious and afraid that a migraine would strike any moment, especially when I was least prepared. But because none of my preheadache symptoms developed into a headache for months, I started to loosen up. I came to expect that my preheadache symptoms were nothing more than a minor discomfort. They did not lead to anything and were well-managed minor migraine symptoms that lasted only 5 minutes.

After the first three months of my treatment, I noticed something else; most of my preheadache symptoms (dizziness , sleepiness, stiffness in my neck, tingling sensation inside my head, and photo- and phonophobia) became less intense.

How Clinicians Measure Success in Preventive Migraine Treatments

A successful preventive treatment for migraines has two features—reduction in both frequency and intensity. After the treatment, the less the migraine attacks and the milder the symptoms during those attacks, the more successful the therapy has been.

As a preventive therapy, my aroma-conditioning was successful. I reduced my migraine attack symptoms— preheadache symptoms became less intense and I completely avoided the headache and postheadache phases.

By the fourth month, my migraine attacks had also started to appear less often. And by six months, I had only 4-5 migraine attacks per month, instead of 4-5 a week. After the first six months, the frequency started to vary. I again had periods with 4-5 migraine attacks per week.

How I Confirmed the Ringing Bell Theory on the Freeway

Because I started to have migraine attacks only once or twice a month and none was likely to develop into a headache, I started to forget my peppermint oil bottle. I used it less and less after the first six months of therapy. One time my wife and I went on a short trip to see some friends. While I was driving on the freeway, I felt a little dizzy and then sleepy. I was about to have a headache, and my wife noticed. She asked me where my peppermint oil bottle was, so she could give it to me. I remembered I didn't have it. Then I thought I would take a few deep breaths through my nose, and imagine I was inhaling fresh peppermint oil. At least I would repeat some of the things I had done when I used the peppermint oil.

I asked my wife to pour some water into a cup. She did, and I dipped the tip of my index finger into the cup, applied the water under and around my nose, as if it had been the oil. I breathed in and out deeply through my nose several times, imagining that I had just inhaled the peppermint oil. Putting water around my nose helped me recreate the experience of the oil. The preheadache disappeared within 5 minutes, and I felt fine.

This could have been one of those rare occasions when I had preheadache without headache. That's why I wouldn't do it again if the peppermint oil was available. But I kept forgetting the oil, especially when I was running errands. I almost forgot I had migraine. I felt sick a couple of times when I didn't have peppermint oil or even water with me. Each time, I was able to prevent my headache phase simply by breathing in and out deeply through my nose, imagining I was inhaling peppermint oil. Usually the preheadaches lasted only five minutes and everything was back to normal. It was great that I could recreate the experience with peppermint oil, minus one more component—the liquid.

But it took more effort and focus on breathing before I felt comfortable. Whenever I had to prevent my headaches with breathing, I felt uncertain and afraid that it might not work. Today I stick to inhaling peppermint oil.

Why did breathing alone or inhaling water prevent my headaches when I had migraine attacks? Let's go back to ringing bell experiment. Using classical conditioning, the man with a white beard taught a dog to salivate upon the ringing of a bell. But he also found that the dog would drool when it heard the sound of a buzzer or the ticking of a metronome, although the dog was never trained to salivate to those stimuli. This is an example of the classical conditioning phenomenon known as stimulus generalization—a reaction to a stimulus similar to another stimulus that has been already conditioned through pairing.

Breathing deeply through my nose and applying water around my nose worked the same way as a ticking metronome or a buzzer when they elicited salivation. Breathing was so similar to the conditioned stimulus—the inhalation of peppermint oil—that it was capable of having the same effect by itself, preventing the headache phase of a migraine attack.

Nonetheless, I didn't use peppermint oil in my therapy only when I forgot the bottle. I felt more confident using the peppermint oil. Plus I enjoyed the smell of peppermint, because it made me feel refreshed.

What to Do When the Effect of the Smell Wears Off

When I had my first headache 12 months after I started my therapy, I became disappointed. Then, I could prevent one headache, but not the next. My headaches tended to get worse. I started having headaches three times a week. At first, I though I did something wrong—maybe I waited too long to inhale the peppermint oil or maybe I didn't breathe enough. But when every preheadache grew to a migraine headache regardless of what I did to prevent it, it was time to rethink everything.

Instead of blaming myself for not doing things correctly, I opened my psychology books to study classical conditioning again. When the man with a white beard stopped pairing the ringing bell with food, his dog started salivating less and less when it heard the bell. In the end the dog no longer drooled at hearing the bell. The same had happened in my experiment. Inhaling peppermint oil gradually reduced its ability to cut short migraine attacks, and ultimately lost its power completely. This phenomenon, when the conditioned stimulus gradually weakens and dies, is called extinction.

Extinction happens when the unconditioned stimulus is no longer paired with the conditioned stimulus. It was thus logical to start pairing inhalation and medicine again. I would become anxious about my headaches and I was afraid that the medicine might not work. But it did. The medicine started preventing the headache phase of my migraine attacks.

I intended to do it exactly as before—pair the unconditioned stimulus (the medicine) with the conditioned stimulus (the peppermint oil) for at least a month. It was a proven system, so why change something that worked. After the sixth pairing, I had preheadache at work and the ergotamine pills weren't in my pocket. Only the peppermint oil was available because I had started keeping a bottle in my car. I inhaled the peppermint oil and it helped—I didn't get a headache. I decided not to use the medicine on my next migraine attack. The peppermint oil helped again. I was back to normal—I had preheadache symptoms that lasted 5 minutes but no headaches.

This time it took me fewer pairings, 6 in two weeks. Twelve months ago, I had needed to pair the medicine and peppermint oil about 20 times. Does this mean that six times is enough for aroma-conditioning to work? I don't know. I can only speculate. If transferring the effect of the drug to the oil needed 20 pairings, the second time I must have experienced a phenomenon known as spontaneous recovery. That is, I did not learn a new behavior but reinforced a previously learned behavior, as the man with a white beard did with his dog. After he extinguished the newly learned behavior of the dog—drooling at a ringing bell, he brought the dog back to the lab in a few days. The man rang the bell and the dog started salivating without any training. The drooling wasn't as intense, but the man could have easily reinforced it by pairing the bell with the food.

The next time the effect of the peppermint oil began to wear off was 19 months later in, May of 2009. This time, I was prepared and recorded every migraine attack and every pairing until shortly after I discontinued the medicine. The first headache I had after those 19 months was on May 26, 2009. After one week and six headaches, I started pairing again.

I paired ergotamine with peppermint oil seven times and then stopped the medicine. Since then I haven't had headaches. Now my migraine attacks are as frequent as three years ago—4-5 times a week, but I don't have headaches.

Experimenting with Other Essential Oils

Bath and Body Works is one of my favorite stores. Because of my success with peppermint, I became interested in aromatherapy and other essential oils. Bath and Body sells a line of essential oils that come in roll-on bottles. You can use the roll-on to apply the oil on your wrists, and then "hold wrists up to nose and breathe in deeply," as the label says. An application of oil on your writs lasts a good hour. I became fond of a blend of vanilla and chamomile—it makes me feel relaxed and I love the smell.

I experimented again. I was risking headaches, but was willing to do it in the name of science. During my next two migraine attacks, I rolled the fresh vanilla-chamomile oil on my writs and inhaled. The headaches did not develop but I felt it took additional breathing until I felt comfortable. The vanilla-chamomile relieved my headaches like the deep breathing without peppermint oil. I enjoyed the smell of vanilla-chamomile essential oil more than the peppermint.

Since that experiment, I've often used the vanilla-chamomile and the peppermint together during migraine attacks. I always inhaled the peppermint first. Both make a better aroma-conditioning medicine: the sure pain relief of peppermint and the added calming effect of vanilla-chamomile blend.

Aroma-Conditioning Doesn't Require Lifestyle Changes

If I had made other changes to my lifestyle besides my aroma-conditioning treatment, it would have been wrong to conclude that the treatment was responsible for my migraine recovery. Had I quit smoking, for example, or cut down on caffeine, my body chemistry would have changed and possibly caused reduction in migraine attacks. It's not that I was careful not to do or take anything that wasn't part of my lifestyle—it just happened. I didn't know then that not changing my

47

lifestyle would help me prove the relationship between my therapy and my improvement.

Except for my treatment, pairing medicine with inhalation, my lifestyle remained the same as before the treatment. I went to bed at the same time of day, didn't start exercising, didn't change my schedule or job, had the same diet and ate at the same time, and had the same amount of coffee and nicotine. Most importantly, I made no extra effort to avoid migraine triggers.

Biological Effects of Aroma-Conditioning

The ringing bell formula can transfer positive, subjective effects like pain relief. It can also transfer negative reactions, as is the case food aversions caused by chemotherapy. Chemotherapy medications can cause negative reactions such as nausea. For example, drinking lemonade before treatment with such medications can transfer the reaction nausea to lemonade. (See Chapter VII, "Drug Effects, the Ringing Bell Theory, and the Mighty Placebo.") Were any negative reactions from my medicine transferred to the peppermint oil? First, I had never experienced any negative reactions from taking ergotamine, i.e. high blood pressure, paleness, numbness, weakness, etc. I had no negative reactions to transfer to peppermint oil.

Expectations in Aroma-Conditioning

Researchers discovered that expectations, in addition to classical conditioning, can influence conditioned drug effects. Both the expectations of the researcher and the expectations of the participants can influence the results of a therapy, because expectations can change the way people act and perceive things. In my aroma-conditioning therapy, I was the researcher and the participant, so when I talk about how expectations influenced my therapy, I have to consider my expectations as a research psychologist and my expectations as a migraine patient.

Sometimes, in their desire to prove their ideas, researches can overlook important facts and emphasize less important facts. The results of an experiment could show that the researcher's ideas were right even if they are not. A researcher might get the results he expected. Results influenced in this way are known as the **experimenter bias effect.**

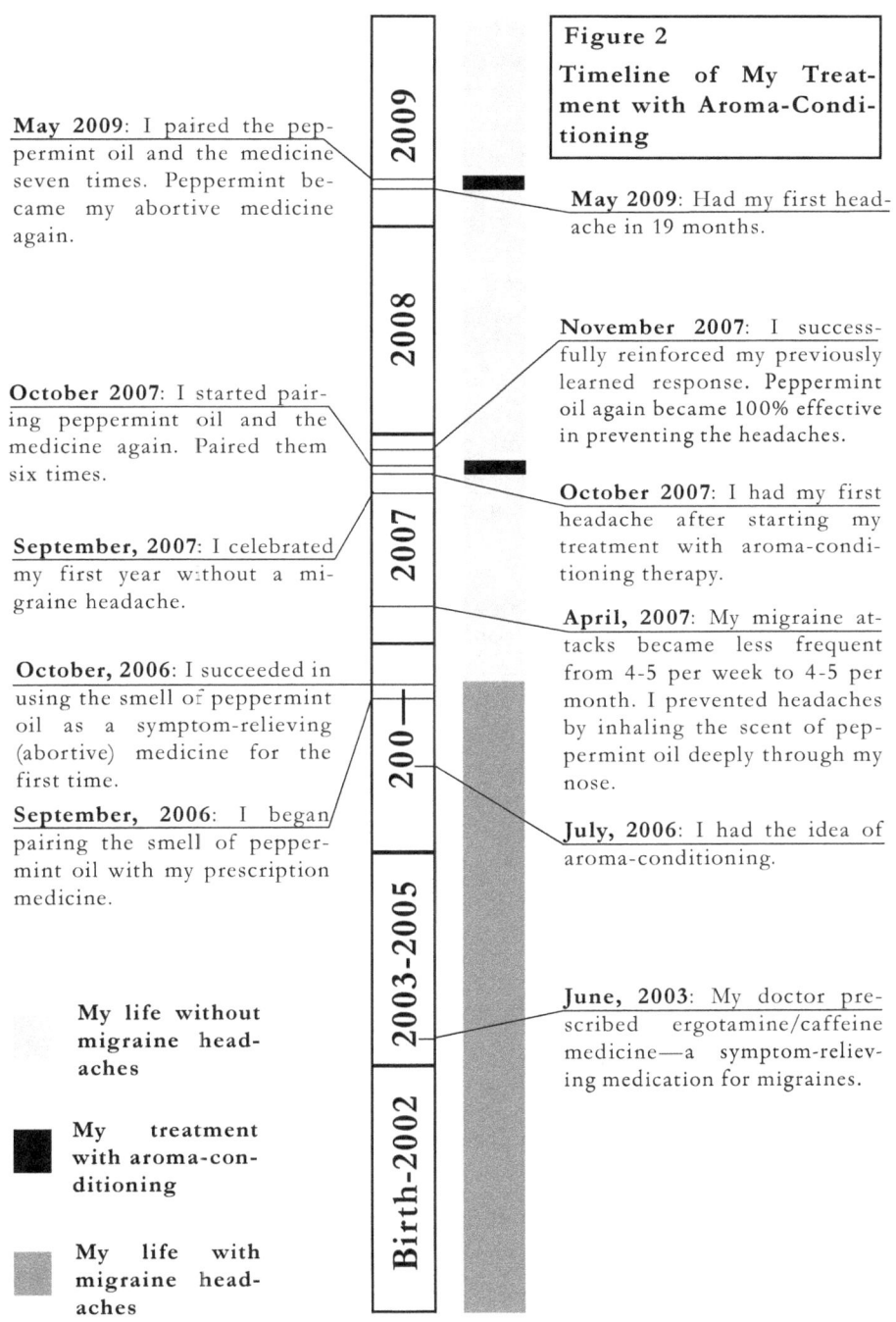

Figure 2
Timeline of My Treatment with Aroma-Conditioning

May 2009: I paired the peppermint oil and the medicine seven times. Peppermint became my abortive medicine again.

May 2009: Had my first headache in 19 months.

November 2007: I successfully reinforced my previously learned response. Peppermint oil again became 100% effective in preventing the headaches.

October 2007: I started pairing peppermint oil and the medicine again. Paired them six times.

October 2007: I had my first headache after starting my treatment with aroma-conditioning therapy.

September, 2007: I celebrated my first year without a migraine headache.

April, 2007: My migraine attacks became less frequent from 4-5 per week to 4-5 per month. I prevented headaches by inhaling the scent of peppermint oil deeply through my nose.

October, 2006: I succeeded in using the smell of peppermint oil as a symptom-relieving (abortive) medicine for the first time.

September, 2006: I began pairing the smell of peppermint oil with my prescription medicine.

July, 2006: I had the idea of aroma-conditioning.

My life without migraine headaches

My treatment with aroma-conditioning

My life with migraine headaches

June, 2003: My doctor prescribed ergotamine/caffeine medicine—a symptom-relieving medication for migraines.

2009
2008
2007
200
2003-2005
2002
Birth-2002

Why am I certain that experimenter bias effect didn't affect the results of my research? Because I had the results of my therapy before I started unraveling the way it worked. I had just learned the basics of classical conditioning and I was a student studying behavioral psychology when I had my idea for the therapy. When I started my therapy, I was driven by my desire to get rid of migraine headaches—not by my desire to prove a hypothesis or gain popularity as an author.

Now let's talk about **my expectations as a migraine patient**. What expectations influenced my therapy the most? Canadian-born psychologist Albert Bandura suggests that there are two kinds of expectations that influence behavior and the outcome of medical treatment. One is **self-efficacy expectancies**—beliefs about one's ability to perform a behavior. The other is **outcome expectancies**—beliefs about the outcome of the behavior. There's research evidence showing that both self-efficacy and outcome expectancies predict patient behavior and treatment outcome.

An example of self-efficacy expectancies are the belief that you can get rid of migraine headaches on your own or that you can successfully apply classical conditioning to treat your migraines. Outcome expectancies are general beliefs about *what will happen if*—like your belief that, in general, classical conditioning can be effective in treating migraines, or that peppermint oil can relieve migraines, or that psychology is a genuine science that can help people with migraines. In principle, the higher your expectancies—whether they are outcome or self-efficacy expectancies, the more likely it is that your treatment will be successful (See Appendix B, "Self-Efficacy.")

To measure my expectations—the ones I felt influenced my therapy, I designed three questionnaires (Appendix C, Figure 11 and Figure 12). The questionnaires measured my attitude, because it must be assumed that attitude predicts expectancies, and a measure of attitude must be proportional to a measure of expectancies. The style of my questionnaires is often used in medical research and health care to measure patient attitudes.

Although my therapy was influenced by non-cognitive, classical learning theory, expectations also play a role in producing a classically conditioned drug effect. I had a certain attitude toward Western medicine, science, and psychology—I valued them highly before I started my therapy. I had high outcome expectancies and believed that Western medicine and science were beneficial for human health.

My other expectancies—self-efficacy expectancies, expectancies specific to my migraine treatment—were low before I started with aroma-conditioning. This could be explained with the fact that I treated my migraines with an approach that had never been tried before. These expectancies increased as my treatment progressed. It is normal to expect that something will have the same effect as before.

I was also and am a person with a strong personal self-efficacy. I am certain I can accomplish the goals I have in life, I view difficulties as challenges, and I attribute my failures to lack of effort. These are beliefs typical for people with high sense of general self-efficacy. Initiating my self-treatment and following through with pairing medicine and peppermint oil also shows my strong sense of self-efficacy.

What did the measure of my expectations mean in relation to aroma-conditioning? It is possible that you need high general self-efficacy expectancies and high outcome expectancies about Western science and medicine. To see how you can improve your sense of self-efficacy, read Chapter V, "Anatomy of Aroma-Conditioning."

Because the sum of my expectations through my aroma-conditioning treatment increased, it is possible that this helped me reduce my anxiety caused by my migraines. I was avoiding a major migraine trigger. The increasing expectations through my therapy are typical of what happens during a successful treatment for a chronic pain disorder. After each successful instance of pain relief, expectations increase. Increased expectations bring more pain relief.

Medicine and Expectations

Medicine relieves pain, and pain relief brings expectations of pain relief, which in turn bring more relief. How do I know that the medicinal effects of ergotamine transferred to the peppermint oil and that peppermint oil relieved my pain? Is it possible that the medicine alone was responsible for my successful treatment? An argument could be made that from the moment I discontinued my medicine, it was the expectations brought by the medicine that improved my symptoms—and not the peppermint oil.

A number of facts prove the peppermint oil prevented my headaches. I used my medicine for two months and discontinued it two weeks before I started the therapy with aroma-conditioning. My headaches returned fully-blown and approximately 10 migraine attacks resulted in a headache. If the medicine was effective in preventing overall migraine symptoms, not just suppressing migraine attacks, my migraines should have improved after those two months. But they didn't.

When I stopped the medicine after my first series of pairings with peppermint oil, the headaches disappeared completely. But I kept having the same number of migraine attacks (4-5 a week), with the same strong preheadache symptoms as before the therapy. I had almost never experienced migraine attacks without the headache phase, which means something had been preventing the headache phases of my migraine attacks when I wasn't using the medicine. The only thing that I was doing to prevent my headaches was inhaling peppermint oil.

Today, almost three years after I started with aroma-conditioning, I still have migraine attacks every month, and often every week. I, however, successfully use peppermint oil to prevent the headaches. I do not take any medicine for my migraines and I do not need to.

Natural History of Illness

Among health care professionals it is well-known that people with chronic pain conditions experience periods of intense pain as well as periods with no pain. Because this phenomenon, one could argue that my migraine management may not have resulted from classical conditioning. Instead it could be argued that just before I started my treatment, my migraine was at its peak and the pain I felt was at its highest intensity.

In fact, throughout my long migraine history, I experienced short and long periods without migraine headaches. The longest period lasted 6 months. But during these periods, I had no migraine attacks, while during my treatment with aroma-conditioning I had migraine attacks, though none developed into headaches.

Prior to my treatment, the periods without migraines appeared at a random. They did not occur in a regular pattern as during my treatment with aroma-conditioning (one year, followed by a short period of therapy, then one and a half years, again followed by a short period of therapy). Another obvious difference is that my longest period without migraines, before I started with aroma-conditioning, was 6 months. I had my first headache one year after I transferred the effect of the drug to the peppermint oil. Headaches started because the conditioned effect of the peppermint oil had started to weaken.

My Migraines after Aroma-Conditioning

Three years after starting my therapy, the frequency of my migraine attacks varies. Sometimes I experience months with almost daily migraine attacks. Other times I have a month without a single migraine attack. None of the migraine attacks develop into a headache—all I feel is the slight discomfort of preheadache symptoms like dizziness, sleepiness, and tingling sensation inside my head. These symptoms go away in about five minutes after I inhale peppermint oil. That I still experience months with frequent migraine attacks after aroma-conditioning is proof that my chronic daily headaches were not rebound headaches.

I had my last migraine attack yesterday, just before completing this book. I was running on the treadmill. Six months ago I started working out regularly. As soon as I felt the tingling sensation inside my head, I applied a few drops of peppermint oil around my nose, breathed in and out a couple of times, then applied the vanilla-chamomile oil roll-on to the inside of my wrists and inhaled several times. It took me about three minutes to cut the migraine attack short, while still running on the treadmill. After achieving a conditioned response, it is as simple as that. Can you compare the debilitating headache with a five minute discomfort?

CHAPTER V

ANATOMY OF
AROMA-CONDITIONING

Outlining Aroma-Conditioning

Aroma-conditioning (from aromatherapy + conditioning) is a migraine
therapy that combines pharmacological drug therapy, behavioral therapy and aromatherapy. On separate migraine attacks aroma-conditioning
acts as an symptom-relieving (abortive) therapy for migraines, but because it reduces the migraine symptoms, it is also preventive. (See Chapter II, "Migraine: More than a Headache.") Aroma-conditioning has one
main goal—to reduce the frequency and intensity of migraine attacks.
Another goal of the therapy is to become drug–free by transferring the
symptom-relieving qualities of a pharmacological drug to something as
safe as the scent of an essential oil.

Inexpensive

Aroma-conditioning is inexpensive. Once the effects of the symptom-
relieving medication are transferred to the essential oil, the only tool
for preventing headaches is a bottle of essential oil, which can cost between 2 and $10 for a small bottle. The contents of a small bottle can be
used to cut short migraine attacks for more than a year.

And if you have an over-the-counter, symptom-relieving medicine that prevents the headache phase of your migraine attacks, then a blister pack of pills might be enough for one series of classical conditioning pairings.

Simple

A closer look at the diagram of aroma-conditioning (page 56) shows how simple the therapy is. A symptom-relieving medicine is taken at the first sign of a migraine attack and paired with an essential oil for a month or slightly longer. The qualities of the medicine transfer to the oil, and then the oil can be used instead of the medicine. The symptom-relieving effects of the aromatherapy oil will eventually weaken. After that, the pairings of medicine and oil must be repeated.

How It Works

There are four main elements required for aroma-conditioning to work: a pharmacological, symptom-relieving medicine that prevents the headache phases of migraine attacks, essential oil of peppermint, classical conditioning, and an appropriate attitude.

Symptom-Relieving (Abortive) Medicine

The medicine must be symptom-relieving, and must effectively prevent the headache phase of a migraine attack. Symptom-relieving medicines for migraines are common over-the-counter analgesics like Aspirin, ibuprofen, and acetaminophen. There are also other, more powerful prescription symptom-relieving medications for migraine. (See Chapter II, "Migraine: More that a Headache.") A symptom-relieving medicine must be used, because the natural response of the medicine—preventing headache phase—allows for classically conditioned drug effects to develop. Classically conditioned drug effects can be achieved deliberately using the famous ringing bell experiment as a model. (See Chapter VI, "The Man with a White Beard.")

Your Expectations

Beliefs in Western Science and Medicine

Beliefs in Classical Conditioning and Psychology

Beliefs in Healing Power of Peppermint and Other Essential Oils

Beliefs that Your Medication Helps

High Sense of Self-Efficacy about Aroma-Conditioning

High Sense of General Self-Efficacy

Start

Read this Book; Educate Yourself about Migraines and Psychology

Use My Experience with Aroma-Conditioning as Model

Find Symptom-Relieving Medicine that Prevents Headache Phase; Talk to Your Doctor

Classical Conditioning

Before Conditioning

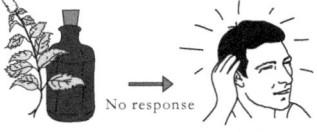
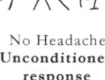

Peppermint Oil
Neutral stimulus

Headache Not Prevented
No Response from Oil

No response · and · Response

Symptom-relieving Medicine
Unconditioned stimulus

No Headache
Unconditioned response

Peppermint oil is a neutral stimulus and cannot prevent the headache phase of a migraine attack. The symptom-relieving medicine is an unconditioned stimulus, and, if taken on time, it can prevent the headache phase.

During Conditioning

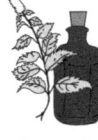
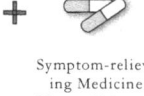
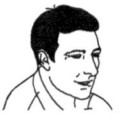

Peppermint Oil
Neutral stimulus

＋

Symptom-relieving Medicine
Unconditioned stimulus

Response

No Headache
Unconditioned response

At the beginning of every migraine attack, peppermint oil is inhaled before the medicine is taken. The medicine prevents headaches while its qualities are gradually transferred to the peppermint oil.

After Conditioning

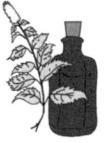

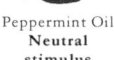
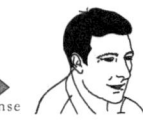

Peppermint Oil
Neutral stimulus

Response

No Headache
Conditioned response

Peppermint oil alone prevents headaches when inhaled at the first signs of a migraine attack. With every prevented headache, sense of self-efficacy and expectations increase, which can make migraine attacks less frequent and less severe.

Figure 3
Basics of Aroma-Conditioning

Peppermint Essential Oil

Peppermint essential oil must be extracted from the stems and leaf of the peppermint plant. Synthetic oil of peppermint may not work as well. Peppermint oil has advantages over other aromatherapy products. It acts as a natural analgesic and anesthetic, relaxes muscles, makes breathing easier, and contributes to a general feeling of relaxation. Peppermint also has a natural ability to relieve migraine symptoms.

Essential Oil Mixtures with Peppermint Oil

Essential oil of peppermint blends well with other essential oils. A mixture of peppermint and say eucalyptus or vanilla oil may be more effective for people who like the smell and taste of eucalyptus or vanilla.

Enjoying something like the smell of vanilla is a conditioned emotional response—a response learned though classical conditioning. Such a response makes you feel relaxed and energized, which can promote natural healing and pain-relief.

Classical Conditioning in Aroma-Conditioning

Classical conditioning is a natural phenomenon; it happens almost everywhere in nature and is a basic way of learning for almost all living organisms. But as the man with a white beard first demonstrated in his lab, conditioning can be deliberately induced. He taught a dog to associate a meal with the ringing of a bell. The dogs natural response to food—drooling—transferred to the ringing bell.

Aroma-conditioning was inspired by the classical conditioning formula. The natural response to an effective symptom-relieving medicine is preventing headache phase of a migraine. Through carefully planned pairing of the symptom-relieving medicine with the smell of peppermint oil, the qualities of the medicine transfer to the smell of peppermint. It is possible that responses to the medicine transfer to other things related to the act of pairing. For example, I was able to prevent a number of headaches by taking deep breaths and imagining I was inhaling peppermint oil.

Which Comes First—Medicine or Aroma?

Theorists say that for classical conditioning to be effective, the initially neutral stimulus (peppermint) must be presented before the unconditioned stimulus (medicine). So according to this, inhaling peppermint oil must precede swallowing of the medicine. But an opposite pairing can also be effective. I conditioned myself by taking the medicine before the peppermint oil.

Pair Medicine and Oil within Seconds

The medicine must follow the inhaling of essential oil within second; classical conditioning is an important evolutionary adaptation that helps organisms prepare for important biological events. Researchers determined that all that is needed for organisms to associate stimuli is one or two seconds. (See Chapter VI, "The Man with a White Beard.")

How to Inhale the Peppermint Oil

Deep, controlled breathing promotes relaxation. Relaxation reduces anxiety and stress that are common migraine triggers. Thus a good practice is using a proven breathing technique while you inhale the essential oil. (See Appendix A, "Proven Self-Help Relaxation Techniques that Work for Migraines.")

Act at the First Signs of a Migraine Attack

When pairing peppermint oil with medicine, it's very important to act quickly at the first signs of a migraine attack. As soon as the first pre-headache symptoms appear, peppermint oil must be inhaled and medicine swallowed. Symptom-relieving medicines work best when taken before the headache starts. If the headache has already started, it is useless to pair the medicine with the essential oil because there won't be a useful response to classically condition.

How Long and How Many Times to Pair Medicine with Oil

There's a scientific irony in aroma-conditioning: a migraine patient who has more frequent migraine attacks has more opportunities to transfer the effects of a medicine. Experimental research showed that the more often the unconditioned and neutral stimuli are paired, the stronger the learning. Thus, the more frequent the headaches, the faster the healing. The first time I tried to classically condition the drug effect of ergotamine, it took me about 20 pairings in one month. It is possible that the number of pairings required might be fewer.

Medicine and Aromatherapy Oil Should Always Be Taken Together

They must. Otherwise the desired response—the essential oil preventing the headache phase during a migraine attack—might take longer to be learned or it might not be learned at all.

Deal with Every Migraine Attack

During aroma-conditioning and after the initial pairings, all migraine attacks must be treated. For example, during a response acquisition phase, having a migraine attack and not taking the medicine and peppermint oil might result in a headache. And learning a response through classical conditioning will take longer or might never be learned.

After the response acquisition phase, after learning to respond to peppermint oil the same way as to the medicine, using the aromatherapy product must become a reflex, just as when you drink water when you are thirsty.

Patient Attitudes and Expectations

Aroma-conditioning was inspired by non-cognitive, behavioral psychology theory. None of my efforts took into account cognitive learning and processes. But not taking those processes into account during the therapy doesn't mean they had no effect. Appropriate attitudes and expectations are a key to every successful therapy, including aroma-conditioning; attitudes predict patient expectations, expectations can change behavior, and behavior influences treatment outcome. The higher your expectations, the more effective your treatment.

If you start your therapy with high outcome expectancies and strong personal self-efficacy expectancies, you will put more effort into your therapy and persist longer. You will take your medicine on time and won't miss opportunities to pair aromatherapy with medicine. You will learn about migraine attack phases and how they work and study classical conditioning. While you are at it, why not learn about your migraine triggers and how to avoid them or master a complimentary relaxation technique, and combine those with aroma-conditioning.

Measure Your Expectations

You can use the two questionnaires from Appendix C to compare the expectations you had before you read this book with the expectations you'll have after you read this book. You can also use the questionnaires to measure your expectations during and after your treatment.

But how can you raise your expectations? A careful reading of this book, which shows the medical evidence that supports aroma-conditioning, may itself increase your outcome expectancies of classical conditioning and aromatherapy. Reading this book can also increase your sense of self-efficacy, or your beliefs about how capable you are in performing specific tasks. You can do this because you are using my success as a model.

Role Models Increase Your Expectations

Modeling is an important concept in the social-learning theory. It is the view that people can learn through observing others. Through modeling, you compare yourself to someone else, your model. When your model succeeds at doing something, your self-efficacy is likely to increase, and vice versa.

Aroma-Conditioning Enhances Your Personal Well-Being and Sense of Accomplishment

Aroma-conditioning is a humanistic, positive approach that, if applied properly, will help a migraine sufferer's life in many ways. Aroma-conditioning helps you gain more self-control and a higher level of self-efficacy. It encourages learning (both in the everyday meaning and the broader sense as understood by psychologists). If you succeed in aroma-conditioning you will emerge from migraines a stronger and more fulfilled person, likely to succeed at everything else.

CHAPTER VI

THE MAN WITH
A WHITE BEARD

Classical conditioning plays an important role in our everyday lives. Think of a sliced lemon, and your mouth will start watering, or consider the pleasure you experience when you think of your favorite vacation destination. Many people have unreasonable fears for snakes or enclosed spaces. All these responses are learned through classical conditioning.

Hamburger Anyone?

The easiest way to demonstrate classical conditioning in real life is taste aversion. Last year, a friend of mine developed a strong taste aversion to hamburgers. She had a double cheeseburger that tasted great and made her full. But after a couple of hours she suddenly had stomach cramps and became nauseated. The cramps and nausea lasted 24 hours. She automatically thought that this was caused by the burger she ate, but it turned out to be the stomach flu. She developed a taste aversion to hamburgers anyway and for one year, just the thought of a hamburger made her feel nauseated.

Many people develop taste aversion the same way, after eating something and becoming sick even if the food and the sickness are unrelated. In taste aversion, food becomes a conditioned stimulus for the symp-

What is Psychology?

Classical conditioning as a form of learning is an important subject of psychology. But what is psychology anyway?

Many people—even well-educated—have misconceptions about psychology; some don't even consider psychology a real science, and those who do usually relate the field only to mental processes and the mind. After explaining how I managed my migraines, I often get comments like these: "I don't underestimate the powers our minds have. I remember that you had problems with headaches and I am glad you have found a way to control your migraines" or "The mind is so powerful; I read that book…"

Today's view of psychology as a discipline related only to mind is influenced by popular culture and the media. It is true that an important aspect of the study of psychology is the mind and mental processes, and early psychologists defined it that way too. But in the early 1900's, a new school of thought called behaviorism developed; it started with the research of the man with a white beard. Behaviorists study observable behavior and learning, so the broader, contemporary definition of psychology is the study of *behavior* and mental processes.

But don't let this pedantic definition fool you. Psychology is a field that offers answers to many exciting questions: How do we learn, feel, forget and remember, and solve problems? What is intelligence, thought, and personality? Why do people tend to develop phobias about snakes and spiders but not about butterflies? Which is more powerful nature or nurture? Why do some medications become more effective after they become popular? (See Chapter VII, "Drug Effects, Classical Conditioning, and the Mighty Placebo.")

Psychology as Science

Psychology is a legitimate field of study, unlike astrology. Though many people believe in it, astrology is a fake science disguised as real science related to astronomy. Astrologists use scientific data and facts from astronomy to prove a false relationship between human destiny and the cosmos. Psychologists, on the other hand, use the scientific method: they observe, collect and analyze information, and make conclusions based on their findings; but more important is that their conclusions are exposed to the possibility to be proven wrong. (See Figure 8 "Steps in the Scientific Method" in Chapter VIII.)

There is also a big difference between psychology as science and popular psychology, also known as pop psychology or pop psych. Popular psychology uses theories and concepts about human behavior that may or may not be based on scientific evidence.

Many self-help books, lectures, newspaper columns, movies, and seminars are based on popular psychology. The term is often used to describe oversimplified and unproven theories about human behavior.

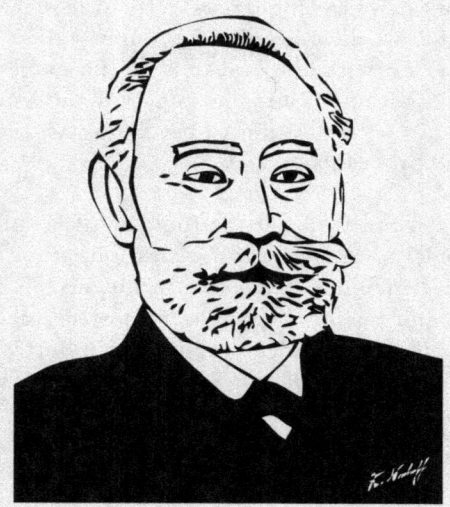

The man with a white beard was Russian scientist **Ivan Pavlov** (1849-1936). Pavlov received a Nobel Prize for his research in the physiology of digestion. But he is better known as the first to describe the classical conditioning phenomenon.

toms caused by an illness. Notice how powerful the conditioning effect is in food aversion; it took my friend only one paring of the hamburger with the stomach flu to develop a food aversion that lasted one year.

On Puppies and Toilet Paper

Through classical conditioning, people learn to respond emotionally to a number of things. Psychologists call this phenomenon conditioned emotional responses. Advertisers, for example, use classical conditioning to make us feel good about products. They pair unconditioned stimuli that produce positive emotions with the products they want us to buy. They try to make us associate positive emotions with the advertised product. One way to achieve this is to use images that create such emotions.

In a television ad for toilet paper, a small puppy—many people adore puppies—appears together with the toilet paper. After seeing the ad many times, the viewers start to associate the brand of toilet paper with the warm feelings created by the image of the puppy. The product becomes conditioned stimulus for the feelings and viewers end up buying the product.

Automatic Negative Reactions

A person can be conditioned to dislike or fear almost anything. Anyone can think of objects, situations, places or people that can make him or her feel upset, frightened, or disgusted.

Say the word Gabrovo to an old classmate of mine and he'll make no secret of his disgust. Gabrovo is the name of the Bulgarian town where we spent our high school years. He had so many negative experiences in Gabrovo that just mentioning the name of that town makes him feel disgusted. In terms of psychology of learning, his negative experiences produced so many negative feelings that the name of the town became a conditioned stimulus that now evokes his negative emotions.

The Little Albert Experiment

The following is one of the most famous and controversial experiments in psychology that would never be allowed today. Psychologists John Watson and graduate student Rosalie Rayner deliberately established a phobia about a white laboratory rat, in an eleven-month old boy known as "Little Albert." After the experiment, Albert's fear of the white rat spread to include white rabbits, cotton wool, and fur coats.

Initially Albert did not show any fear of the white rat: "White rat suddenly taken from the basket and presented to Albert. He began to reach for rat with left hand" (Watson & Rayner, 1920). But Albert, like most children, was afraid of loud noises. During the experiment, whenever Little Albert tried to reach the rat, Watson made a loud noise by hitting a steal bar with a hammer. After only seven times of pairing the loud noise with the rat, the child developed a phobia—he was terrified by the presence of the rat alone. The instant Albert saw the rat, he cried, and tried to crawl away as quickly as possible.

Afraid of Rabbits

Phobias, however, can be unlearned through a process called counter-conditioning, or systematic desensitization (See Figure 2.) In counter-conditioning, an unwanted response, like fear, is replaced by another response incompatible with the unwanted response. Psychologist Mary Cover Jones helped a three-year-old boy named Peter overcome his fears of white rabbits. Peter was also afraid of cotton, fur coats, and feathers.

Jones paired the presence of the rabbit with a pleasant feeling for Peter—eating candy. While Peter was eating his favorite candy, Jones brought the rabbit into the room and kept it "as close as she could without" making Peter nervous (Jones, 1924, p. 466). Every day, Jones brought the rabbit closer and closer to Peter. She also let other kids play with the rabbit while Peter was watching. Eventually, Peter was not only cured of his phobia, but he also got to like the rabbit. Peter's fear of other objects like fur coats and cotton was also gone. He learned a new response—enjoying the presence of the rabbit.

Before Conditioning

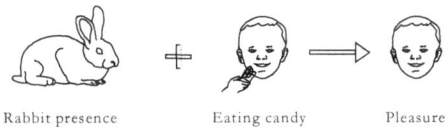

Rabbit presence → Fear and Eating candy → Pleasure

Before conditioning, the presence of the rabbit terrifies Peter and eating candy makes him experience pleasure.

During Conditioning

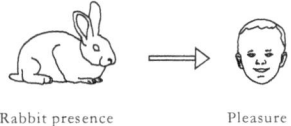

Rabbit presence + Eating candy → Pleasure

During conditioning the presence of the rabbit is paired with pleasant experience—eating candy. With each pairing, Peter started feeling more and more comfortable with the presence of the rabbit.

After Conditioning

Rabbit presence → Pleasure

After conditioning, Peter was happy to see the rabbit. The new response (pleasure) was incompatible with Peter's original response at the presence of the rabbit—fear.

Figure 4
Counterconditioning—the Experiment with Peter
Figure demonstrates how Dr. Jones helped a 3-year-old boy unlearn his unreasonable fear of rabbits

Other Elements of the Ringing Bell Theory

Response Acquisition

Classical conditioning is a process starting with a phase called response acquisition. During this phase, the unconditioned stimulus and conditioned stimulus are paired. Each pairing is called a trial. But the strength of a learned behavior has limits. Although initially the probability of the conditioned response (to appear after the conditioned stimulus) increases significantly with each pairing, once this limit is reached the strength of the response remains the same, no matter how many times you pair the conditioned stimulus with the unconditioned stimulus.

Extinction

In classical conditioning, extinction occurs when the conditioned response gradually weakens or disappears. This can happen when the conditioned stimulus (ringing bell) is repeatedly presented without the unconditioned stimulus (food). After Pavlov taught his dog to salivate upon hearing a bell, he started another experiment: He had his dog hear the bell without presenting the food. As a result, the dog gradually decreased the amount of salivation until the ringing bell no longer made the dog drool.

> **Higher-order Conditioning**
>
> When a conditioned stimulus is paired with a new neutral stimulus, a higher-order conditioning may happen. A classic example of higher-order conditioning is a dog learning to drool at a flashing light after pairing the flashing light with an already conditioned stimulus like a ringing bell that makes the dog drool.

Spontaneous Recovery

Pavlov's dog was brought back to the laboratory days after he extinguished its learned behavior. But as the researcher sounded the bell again, the dog started salivating. Although the conditioned response, salivation, was not as strong as before, it did reappear without training. The reappearance of the conditioned response, called spontaneous recovery, showed that the learned behavior still existed after extinction.

Stimulus Generalization

Stimulus generalization is a reaction to a stimulus similar to the conditioned stimulus. Pavlov, for example, trained his dog to salivate to a high-pitched tone. He found that the dog salivated even if he sounded a higher tone without ever pairing the higher tone with the sight of food.

Pavlov also noticed that his dog would salivate not only to ringing of a bell but also to other similar sounds like ticking of a metronome or the sound of a buzzer.

Stimulus Discrimination

Let's say that you conditioned your dog to salivate to the sound of a ringing bell. You discover, like Pavlov, that your dog now salivates to your cell phone ringing. But if you repeatedly pair the ringing bell with the food, and sound your cell phone without presenting the food, your dog will eventually learn to discriminate between the sound of the bell and the ring tone of your cell phone; your dog will salivate to the bell but not to the ring tone. This is called stimulus discrimination.

Biological Preparedness and Counterpreparedness

Species are biologically prepared to learn association between certain stimuli and responses. Phobias and taste aversion are good examples. Humans readily develop phobias for snakes and spiders, but almost never from rabbits, stones, or shoes. Similarly, humans are biologically prepared to associate sickness with food and taste, rather than sights and sounds. The reason is that fear of snakes and spiders and readiness to associate sickness with food has been helping us survive, especially during our evolutionary past.

Making the Most of a Ringing Bell

Time Between Neutral and Conditioned Stimulus

Learning through classical conditioning is most effective when the neutral stimulus is presented right before the unconditioned stimulus—usually in an interval of no more than a couple of seconds. (See Figure 5.) That is, one stimulus should accurately predict the appearance of another. The reason for this is because classical conditioning is a genetic adaptation that prepares organisms for important physiological events. In Pavlov's experiments, the ringing of a bell signaled the appearance of food and the dog salivated because it prepared to eat.

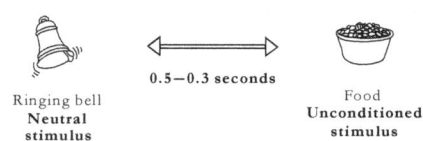

Figure 5
Interval between Stimuli
The most effective interval between the neutral stimulus and the unconditioned stimulus is no more than a few seconds.

Always Pair the Conditioned Stimulus and the Unconditioned Stimulus

At the beginning, it is very important for the conditioned stimulus to always appear together with the unconditioned stimulus. Presenting both stimuli only some of the times would greatly inhibit the learning process. This rule changes after the conditioned response is established.

Time between Each Pairing

Classical conditioning is most effective when the time between each pairing is equally and moderately spaced. (See Figure 6.) For more effective learning, conditioned and unconditioned stimuli should be paired at even intervals. The more uneven are the intervals between each pairing, the more time it will take to achieve a classically conditioned response.

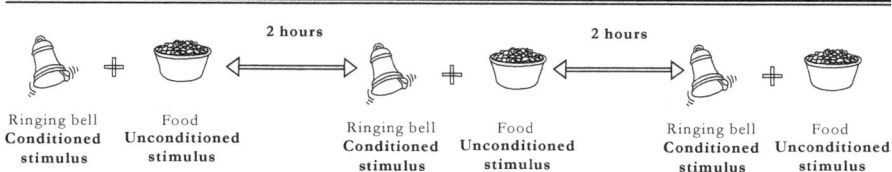

Figure 6
Time between Each Pairing
Classical conditioning is more effective when parings are equally and moderately spaced.

How Often to Pair

The number of times a conditioned stimulus is paired with an unconditioned stimulus is also important. The more these two are paired, the more effective learning is.

Stronger Stimulus, Stronger Response

Generally speaking, a stronger stimulus produces stronger response; a siren, for example, will produce a stronger conditioned response than a ringing bell. In clinical placebo effect studies (more on placebo in the next chapter), patients who receive a drug through injections develop stronger responses than those who take the drug in the form of pills. (See Chapter VII, "Drug Effects, the Ringing Bell Theory, and the Mighty Placebo.")

Is There a Maximum Effect of Classical Conditioning?

Learning does not increase indefinitely. In the beginning, the strength of learning greatly increases with each pairing. The strength of learning is the ability of unconditioned stimulus, like food, to produce a conditioned response, like salivation. But eventually, the strength of learning reaches a maximum and remains constant—even if the conditioned stimulus and conditioned response are still paired.

Mind Your Behavior

"Give me a dozen healthy infants, well-formed, and my own speci-
fied world to bring them up in and I'll guarantee to take any one
at random and train him to
become any type of specialist I might select —doctor,
lawyer, artist, merchant-chief
and, yes, even beggar-man and
thief, regardless of his talents,
penchants, tendencies, abili-
ties, vocations, and race of his
ancestors. I am going beyond
my facts and I admit it, but so
have the advocates of the contrary and they have been doing it for many thousands of
years" (Watson 1930, p.82).

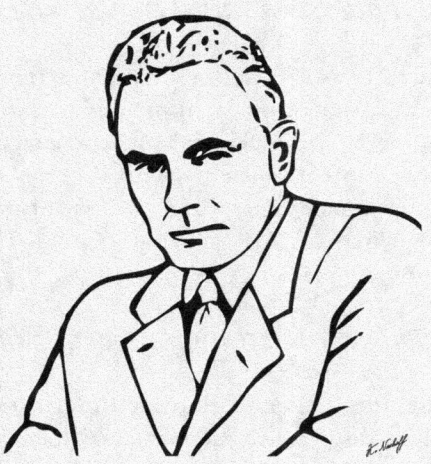

This famous quote by John
Watson demonstrates his view
on nature vs. nurture debate, from a perspective in psychology called
behaviorism. Another important name of this school of though is
American behaviorist B.F. Skinner, who wrote Walden Two (1948), a
controversial but important book about a utopian society founded on
behaviorist principles. Behaviorism remained most popular among
American psychologists like Watson and Skinner, but it originated
from the work of Ivan Pavlov.

Behaviorism, also known as the learning perspective in psychology, is
the main point of view in this book; aroma-conditioning is founded
upon behaviorist principles. Behavioral psychology deals with how
the environment shapes behavior and how behavior is acquired, reinforced, or discouraged by environmental forces. Behaviorists also
rely on observable and measurable behavior rather than on what's
going on in people's minds.

Although behaviorism has many critics, its approach—using observable behavior, one noted through the senses—helped the whole field

of psychology establish itself as a legitimate science. As opposed to mental processes like feelings and intentions, observable behavior can be easily measured and the collected data can be used in research.

Classical Conditioning and the Psychological Perspectives

Classical conditioning was initially subject of behavioral psychologists. But as knowledge about learning grew, psychologists discovered that classical conditioning can be influenced by other factors. Evolutionary psychologists, for example, emphasize that certain survival traits, like fear of snakes, play a great role in classical conditioning. On the other hand, cognitive psychologists proved that in many cases expectations, at least in humans, influence classical conditioning. Cognitive psychologists also see classical conditioning as a mechanism to predict events from the environment.

CHAPTER VII

DRUG EFFECTS, THE RINGING
BELL THEORY, AND
THE MIGHTY
PLACEBO

You've seen how conditioning plays an important role in our everyday lives, and that conditioning can be used by psychologists to treat psychological problems like phobias. Here you'll learn how conditioning can be used as treatment for physiological problems.

Decaf and Black Coffee Can Make You Feel the Same?

To understand how drug effects can become classically conditioned, consider the following example about caffeine and coffee. Researchers found that decaf and black coffee can both make you feel the same, if you are a regular coffee drinker. In one study, regular coffee drinkers had decaf coffee, believing they were given regular black coffee. Yet, the coffee drinkers experienced the physiological and psychological sensations produced by caffeine in black coffee (Flaten & Blumenthal, 1999, as cited by Mikalsen, Bertelsen, & Flaten, 2001). How did this happen?

Coffee drinkers had learned to associate the smell and taste of coffee with the pleasant effects of caffeine in black coffee. With every cup of coffee, the smell and taste of coffee are paired with caffeine until the smell and taste alone are able to produce the effects of caffeine.

Before Conditioning

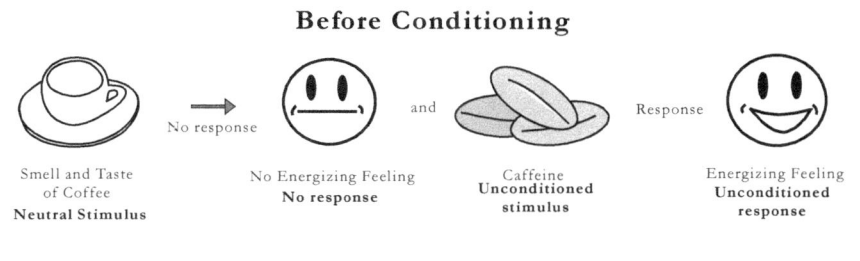

| Smell and Taste of Coffee **Neutral Stimulus** | No Energizing Feeling **No response** | Caffeine **Unconditioned stimulus** | Energizing Feeling **Unconditioned response** |

During Conditioning

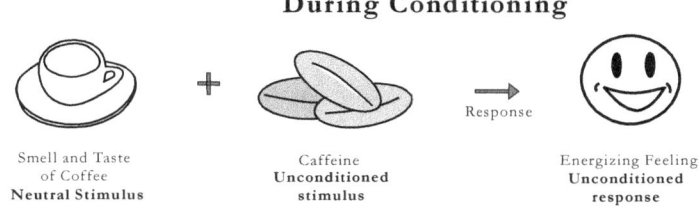

| Smell and Taste of Coffee **Neutral Stimulus** | Caffeine **Unconditioned stimulus** | Energizing Feeling **Unconditioned response** |

After Conditioning

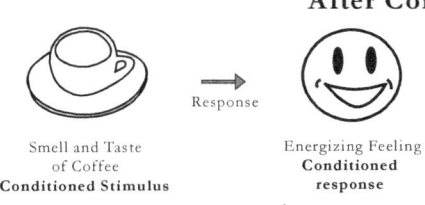

| Smell and Taste of Coffee **Conditioned Stimulus** | Energizing Feeling **Conditioned response** |

Figure 7
Classical Conditioning and Caffeine

Another example of how drug effects become classically conditioned is food aversion as a result of chemotherapy drugs. Food eaten before the therapy becomes conditioned stimulus for unpleasant reactions of the chemotherapy drugs—reactions such as nausea and vomiting. This makes people less likely to eat the food that was previously paired with chemotherapy. In one clinical study, children ate ice cream just before chemotherapy with drugs known to cause nausea and vomiting. The children developed aversion to ice cream that lasted for weeks.

The Ringing Bell Theory and the Immune System

Ivan Pavlov was the first who proposed that the effects of a drug could be classically conditioned: the curing properties of a drug could be transferred to something harmless, like a ringing bell, sense of smell or taste. Say you successfully pair a neutral stimulus like a ringing bell with a drug used for treating a physiological illness; the harmless ringing bell will become the instrument of the treatment.

After Pavlov, psychologist Robert Ader and immunologist Nicholas Cohen discovered that classical conditioning can affect the immune system. Ader used laboratory rats to study taste aversion when he decided to pair sweetened water with a drug that, as it turned out, suppressed the immune system of the rats. After a number of pairings, the sweetened water alone suppressed the immune system of the rats.

The drug whose properties Ader transferred to the sweetened water was cyclophosphamide—a powerful chemotherapy drug that is used, in humans, for treating autoimmune disorders and various types of cancer. When used for autoimmune disorders, suppressing the immune system is actually the desired effect.

Autoimmune disorders cause a person's immune system to attack the body's own cells, tissues, and organs. Although immune-suppressing drugs, like cyclophosphamide, can help suppress the harmful effects of the immune system disorders, the drugs themselves have dangerous side-effects: they can damage the liver, bone marrow, and even cause cancer. And because of the results in animal studies, researchers believe that the same will work for humans—pair the immune-suppressing drug with a sense of smell or taste, then use the smell or taste instead of the drug.

The Mighty Placebo

For a long time the placebo effect has been looked down on by many in the medical field. Today, the placebo effect is of great interest to psychologists and health practitioners. The reason is that the placebo effect has been proven to have a real medical value.

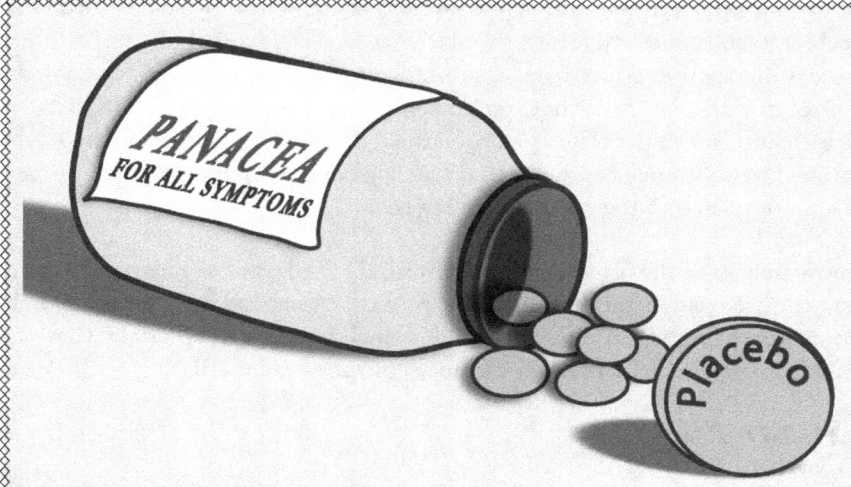

Panacea for All Symptoms

Although a little extreme, the following statement has a lot of truth: The history of medicine is the history of placebo effect.

Placebo effect is a phenomenon in which classical conditioning plays a key role. Considering recent scientific literature and discoveries, it appears that placebo effect might be involved in all forms of a medical treatment. For example, researchers found that your beliefs in the curing power of a drug, your doctor's qualifications, or the legitimacy of the treatment, makes that drug, doctor or treatment more effective in helping you overcome an illness—no matter how relevant that treatment is.

Various psychoactive drugs have become more effective after their introduction, and many specialists attribute this to placebo phenomenon; people's confidence in those drugs has increased and therefore the effectiveness of the drugs also increased.

The placebo effect is a physiological or psychological effect, produced by a treatment or substance, but that is not the result of any special property of that treatment or substance. A placebo is a treatment or substance that has no special property in producing physiological or psychological effect. The placebo effect need not to be health-related. In fact, classically conditioned drug effects like the example of coffee and caffeine, can be described as the placebo effect.

However, for the purpose of this book we'll talk about health-related, medicinal placebo effect. In medical terms, the placebo effect is the psychological or physiological therapeutic effect from a substance or treatment, but that is not the result of any special medicinal (pharmacological) properties of the substance or treatment. In health-related placebo effect, produced at medical settings, the treatment or substance can have pharmacological properties but these properties are not related to the condition being treated.

Some instances of the placebo effect are desirable and positive like reduced pain or swelling. Negative, unwanted instances of the placebo effect (like increase in pain or worsening of a condition) are sometimes called nocebo effect. Classical conditioning is involved in many instances of the placebo effect.

A Sugar Pill

Consider the following archetypal case of the placebo effect. A medical researcher prescribes a patient an active painkiller drug in the form of a pill. After several instances of taking the drug in the same medical environment, the researcher exchanges the drug with a sugar pill. The patient is unaware that the pill is actually sugar disguised as a pharmacological drug. Nevertheless, the patient feels better and reports that the pain has disappeared. Here, the placebo is the drug and the placebo effect is the reduced pain. Although the placebo sugar pill has no special power to produce pain relief, it actually does.

Two main theories in psychology are used to explain the placebo effect phenomenon—classical conditioning, from the learning perspective in psychology, and expectancy theory, from the cognitive perspective. In addition, biological psychology gives important objective evidence for the placebo effect.

Placebo and the Ringing Bell Theory

A behavioral psychologist, for example, might say that the archetypal medicinal placebo effect described above results from classical conditioning: the sight and sound of the medical setting, the room, the doctors, the nurses, and the act of taking the pill all become conditioned stimuli for the conditioned response pain relief. These stimuli have been previously paired with the pharmacological drug—the unconditioned stimulus. Notice that the sights, sounds and the rest together with the fake drug are the placebo and the conditioned response (pain relief) is the placebo effect.

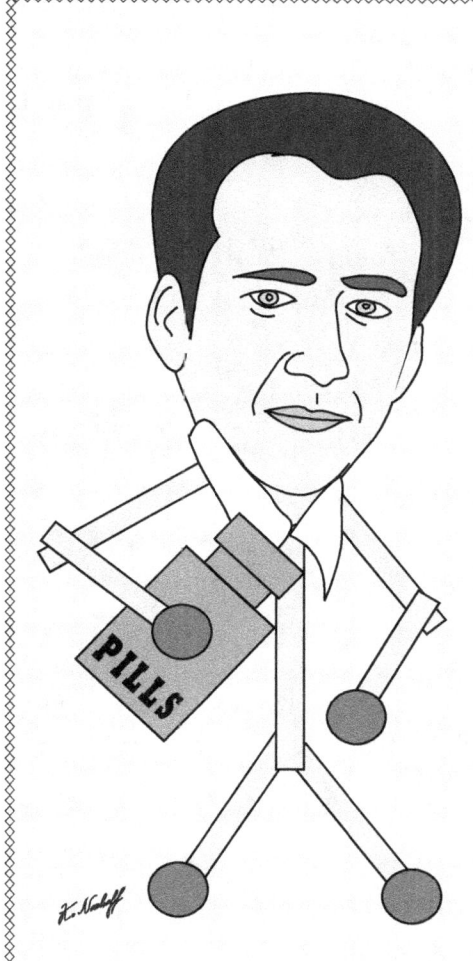

Matchstick Men: Classical Placebo in the Movies

Have you seen Nicolas Cage in the movie Matchstick Men (2003)? In the movie, the main character Roy (Cage), a professional con man, suffers from a number of psychological disorders: obsessive-compulsive disorder, panic attacks, agoraphobia, and Tourette's syndrome. Roy goes to a fake psychiatrist who gives him a fake drug disguised as a real psychoactive drug. Roy's symptoms improve even though the pills he's been taking are vitamins.

Though fictional, the story demonstrates the classical placebo effect that results from expectancies rather than classical conditioning. It is Roy's trust in the health care professional, the treatment, and the drug that made him feel better. And no pharmacological drug was involved.

Scientists have demonstrated that the placebo effect can result from non-conscious learning through classical conditioning, without conscious expectations. Researchers conditioned clinical patients with buprenorphine—a drug that slows down and reduces breathing (Benedetti et al., 1998; Benedetti, Amanzio, et al., 1999 as cited by Stewart-Williams & Podd, 2004). The effect of the drug before conditioning was mild and the patients didn't notice it. The researches, however, were able to measure the effect.

Because the patients did not notice the effect of the drug, they did not have any conscious expectations of any effect after conditioning. But after conditioning, the placebo disguised as buprenorphine caused slowness and reduction in breathing, while patients were still unaware of the physical effects that the placebo produced.

Placebo and Expectations

A cognitive psychologist could argue that the patient's health at the archetypal placebo effect improves because of his conscious expectancies for getting better. The patient's belief in the power of the pill or medical treatment, his relationship with and trust in the doctor, his experience with Western medicine, and his general life experience could all have shaped his conscious expectations. A review of literature on the role of conscious expectancies in the placebo effect showed that expectancies can improve symptoms in the form of "improved mood, less anxiety, reduced pain" and they can also improve a "patient's disease status (e.g. lowered blood pressure, immunological changes, and better metabolic control)" (Crow et al., 1999, p. iii).

> **Expectations or Expectancies**
>
> Researchers prefer the technical words *expectancy* and *expectancies* when they in fact discuss expectations—what you think or hope will happen.
>
> Though I can't force myself say *expectancy* when it simply means expectation, I can't avoid the word completely because *expectancy* is embedded in the cognitive theory about human behavior.

There is evidence in the placebo field that demonstrates that the placebo effect can be produced by conscious expectancies alone, without classical conditioning. In several placebo studies in humans, study participants were given the same placebo but were "told to expect opposite effects" (Stewart-Williams & Podd, 2004, p. 335). The participants reported different effects from the same placebo so researcher attributed these effects to the verbally-induced expectations of the participants (Stewart-Williams & Podd, 2004, p. 335).

Behavioral-Cognitive Model of the Placebo Effect

In fact, evidence suggests that both expectancies and classical conditioning—among other factors like observational learning, memory, self-efficacy, the body's own painkiller system, level of motivation, and desire for recovery—

shape the placebo effect. Although there are instances when the placebo effect was entirely produced by either classical conditioning or expectations, it is likely that, in most cases, both are involved. Let's go back to the archetypal placebo effect example above to see how.

The patient's expectancies might be involved even before the treatment starts: his general experience with Western medicine, his memory and intelligence capacity, his education, his relationship with the doctor, and his knowledge about the effectiveness of the drug could have contributed to his conscious expectations about the treatment. On the other hand, classical conditioning, which involves automatic non-conscious processes, can cause the development of more expectations. After several pairings, the patient expects that after taking the sugar pill his pain will go away. The pain relief that results from conditioning can increase the patient's expectations of relief, and therefore contribute to an even stronger placebo effect.

Generally, supporters of either theory accept that expectancy and conditioning play a role in the placebo effect. Scientists, however, disagree on how important those roles are compared to each other. Some believe that in humans expectations are more important than conditioning when it comes to the placebo effect. This view is supported by recent studies that demonstrate the underlying relationship between placebo and expectations in humans, especially in the placebo pain relief.

Hidden injections of pain killers like morphine, injected by computer-controlled machines without doctors or nurses present, were less effective in producing pain relief than injections given by medical personnel (Amanzio & Benedetti, 1999). This demonstrates how important expectations of pain relief are in producing actual pain relief. Why are expectations important for humans? It is possible that the higher an organism stands in the evolutionary ladder, the more important the role of expectations and cognition are. Evidence for the placebo effect that was influenced by expectations is more common in placebo field research.

Objective Evidence for the Placebo Effect

The measured physiological changes from placebo, which is the biological perspective in psychology, give scientific grounds for accepting the placebo effect as a legitimate form of treatment. These effects are objective, physiological—not subjective effects like reports of reduced pain.

Placebos involved in placebo pain relief, for example, don't have the pharmacological properties of painkiller drugs, but they activate the body's natural painkiller system. Placebo pain relief can often result from release of endorphins in the brain.

In a landmark study, researchers compared the brain area activated by a powerful opioid, remifentanil, with the area activated by a placebo saline (Petrovic et al., as cited by Koshi & Short, 2007). The study participants received the placebo after the drug. Because of the unusual similarity of the activated areas, scientists concluded that placebo pain relief stimulates the release of endorphins and activates the body's pain killer system just like opioid drugs do.

If I Your Doctor Says It Works, It Works

There's evidence suggesting that some physiological systems are influenced by conscious processes while others are influenced by conditioned unconscious processes (Benedetti, 2006). Expectations override the effects of conditioning when expectations of pain relief are influenced by verbal information—like the doctor telling the patient that the drug will be effective or ineffective.

But expectations influenced by verbal information do not affect the classically conditioned placebo effects of an "increase or decrease of growth hormone and cortisol" (Benedetti, 2006, p. s101). "If pre-conditioning is carried out with migraine medicine sumatriptan, which stimulates growth hormone and inhibits cortisol secretion, a significant increase of growth hormone and decrease of cortisol blood concentrations can be found after placebo administration, even though opposite verbal suggestions are given" to patients (Benedetti, 2006, p. s101).

Differences between Aroma-Conditioning and Clinical Treatments with Placebos

Shift in Control

Shift in control is the obvious difference between aroma-conditioning and the archetypal clinical placebo effect. In the clinical placebo effect, doctors and researchers control and plan the treatment. But with aroma-conditioning, the patient is the one taking the active role. The patient plans and carries out the treatment and keeps track of the progress.

Aroma-conditioning is classical conditioning, a behavioral therapy. Behavioral therapies are used by psychologists to treat patients. But again the difference between a typical behavioral therapy and aroma-conditioning is the shift in control. The one receiving the classical conditioning treatment, the patient, is the one applying it.

Complete Lack of Deception

Most instances of the clinical placebo effect involve some form of deception—giving a fake substance or treatment that the researcher or doctor knows has no pharmacological effect. Aroma-conditioning doesn't involve deception; just the opposite—gaining knowledge. This makes aroma-conditioning an ethical therapy. Ethics in experimental psychology and medicine in general have always been and will continue to be a central issue. Just think of some of the most famous experiments in psychology like the Little Albert Experiment—such experiments are impossible to conduct today because of ethics.

CHAPTER VIII

MIGRAINE SCIENCE

I used the scientific method in my migraine experiment (Figure 8). The method involved developing a hypothesis and setting up an experiment. But how a research psychologist like Pavlov sets about doing science with the scientific method?

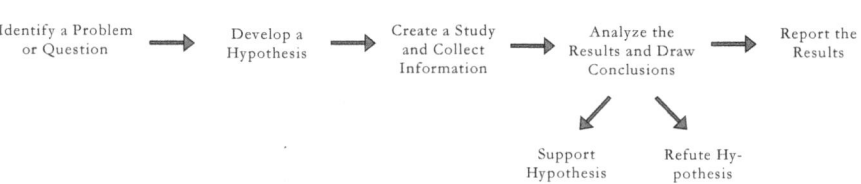

Figure 8
Steps in the Scientific Method

How I Turned My Idea into a Scientific Experiment

An interesting idea, based on observation, may prompt a researcher to ask a question: The dog drools when it hears my footsteps—is it possible to teach the dog to drool when it hears a ringing bell? Drug effects can be classically conditioned—what might happen if a powerful migraine drug was paired with something safe, a specific smell or taste? Many prescription drugs for migraine can suppress headaches, but using them regularly can lead to serious side effects. One such drug is ergotamine, which helps me prevent my headaches right now. Will classical conditioning work for my migraine or it does with other disorders?

Questions like these can be turned into a hypothesis: *A person with migraine can be conditioned to respond to a safe stimulus, like smelling or tasting something pleasant, the same way that person responds to an effective medicine.* In other words, transfer the relief caused by a medicine to a particular smell or taste. Then use the smell or taste in place of the medicine. (See Figure 9a.)

This was my first hypothesis, but it wasn't specific enough. I had a drug in mind, ergotamine, and I needed to choose a smell or taste. I chose the smell of mint oil. So, this is what scientists call a working hypothesis, the one that allowed me to put my ideas into practice:

A person with migraine headaches who prevents his headache phase from developing using ergotamine/caffeine medicine can be conditioned to respond to the smell of mint oil the same way he responds to the ergotamine/caffeine medicine.

Scientific Hypothesis: a statement or idea that can be tested for true or false. A hypothesis must be able to be supported or refuted through testing.

Working Hypothesis: A working hypothesis is a hypothesis about something specific, something that can be tested in practice.

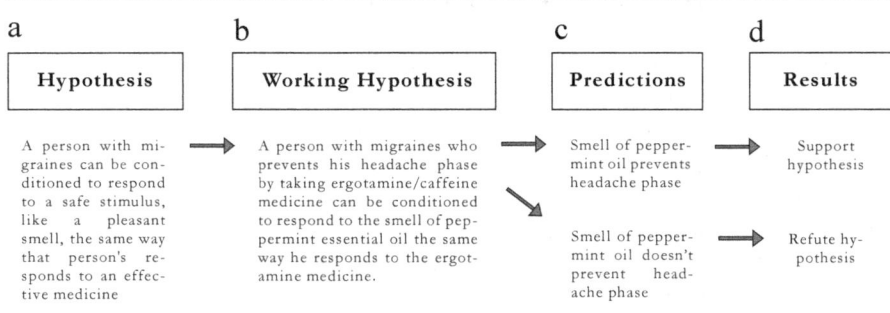

Figure 9
My Idea for Migraine Therapy in Scientific Terms
You can see how my general idea about a migraine therapy evolved into
something specific. I decided to test it.

The Las Vegas Experiment

My idea to devise an experiment came
from my reading of Pavlov. Collecting
evidence on classical conditioning re-
lies on the experimental method. This
method is still used by psychologists and
clinical researchers.

In everyday life, people experiment without realizing it. For example, suppose you
enter a Las Vegas hotel suite you reserved
last week. The minute you put your bag

Experimental Method

A research method psychologists and other scientists use
to find out how the changes
in one thing (the independent variable) affects another
(the dependent variable).

on the floor you want to turn on the lights. You notice the two identical switches on your left side, and you turn one of them on. But the
switch starts the air conditioner—not the lights. Your "hypothesis"
was that the first switch would turn on the lights, which proved to
be wrong. Now you turn on the other switch and the lights come on.
You conducted another experiment and confirmed your hypothesis. In
both experiments, you manipulated a switch to see if it would cause the
lights to turn on. In the second experiment, you found a cause-and-
effect relationship.

Psychologists similarly look for cause-and-effect relationships in their experiments. However, instead of manipulating something trivial like a switch, they manipulate something about a person or a lab animal (study participants). Psychologists want to see if their actions caused the participants to behave differently.

Ringing Bell and Wagging Tail

A hypothesis predicts a cause-and-effect relationship between two or more things. The cause is called the independent variable and the effect, the dependent variable. In the Las Vegas experiment, the independent variable is the turning on of the light switch, and the dependent is the lights being on.

Research psychologists manipulate the independent variable to see if it causes changes in the dependent variable. In Pavlov's famous experiment, the pairing the ringing bell with food is the independent variable and the salivation of the dog is the dependent variable. The ringing bell causes the salivation.

It is also common for psychological experiments to have more than one independent variable. It's possible that Pavlov's dog started wagging its tail when in heard the bell ringing because it knew that food was coming. The wagging tale is another effect of the independent variable—pairing a ringing bell with food.

In my experiment, the independent variable was the treatment—learning through classical conditioning measured in the pairing mint oil and a drug. The effect, or dependent variable, was mint oil serving as medicine (the smell of mint preventing the headache phase from developing. I measured how many times mint oil prevented the development of the headache phase of my migraines without using medicine.

Foretold is Forearmed

I saw the future of my experiment in black and white. I though that if my experiment resembled these of Pavlov, Watson, and Cover Jones, mint oil would work the same way as the drug or my conditioning would be fruitless and nothing would happen. I had never heard anyone try this for migraine before. If it worked, I would have a harmless substitute for my powerful drug, and I wouldn't have to worry about side effects, even if I used the oil every day.

Scientists also make predictions about what will happen when they apply their hypotheses. They try to predict what will happen if their hypothesis is right and what will happen if their hypothesis states a relationship that doesn't exist.

Am I Cousins with Norman Cousins?

Many experiments in psychology are used to determine whether a particular treatment or substance causes improved health. But most experiments involve more than one person as a study participant. For a time, I was skeptical about my achievement. I was afraid that one day a licensed medical researcher would dismiss my migraine therapy as an argument by anecdote—a logical fallacy meaning that you base your argument solely on one example.

An example of argument by anecdote is the premise of a best seller self-help book by author and journalist Norma Cousins. Cousins argued that he recovered from a terminal illness by taking extremely high doses of vitamin C, and by making himself laugh watching his favorite comedies. Cousin's arguments in *Anatomy of an Illness as Perceived by the Patient: Reflections on Healing* (1979) are dismissed by psychology textbook authors as argument by anecdote. I wanted to compare my experiment with Cousins's self-help. Cousins's ideas didn't originate from a scientific theory. Alternative medicine may cause health improvement because of the placebo effect phenomenon.

On the other hand, aroma-conditioning came from an established scientific theory—classical conditioning. The scientific method was used, and my experiment resembled those of Watson and Jones. Both used only one participant in their experiments and these were two of the most famous experiments in psychology. (See Appendix D, " Jones's Experiment with Peter vs. My Experiment with Aroma-Conditioning.")

In my experiment, the researcher and the participant were the same person. What would be the difference if say a psychologist said "Do this and that, and record your experience for me. Do you feel any improvement now? In medical research, the patients often take the role of researcher by keeping diaries to record symptom history and the results of treatment. This is especially important for patients suffering from chronic conditions, such as migraine headaches.

Watson and Jones did research that was qualitative, dealing with subjective things like fear. They didn't need to measure Peter's and Little Albert's blood pressure to see that the children were afraid; crying can be a sure sign of fear in children. My experiment involved qualitative description than number crunching. Headaches, like fear, are subjective. Although, in most cases, we can't measure extreme migraine headaches with numbers, we can say for sure when someone is in extreme pain and describe this using language instead of numbers.

The Approach of Watson and Jones in Their Research

The researchers used the experimental method, but each of them included only one participant. This approach to research is known as the single-case study design. Medical researchers use single-case studies to test a current theory, expand on it, or challenge it, as is in the cases of Watson and Jones's experiments. In this type of single-case designs, depending on the purpose, the researcher may choose a participant who is typical or unique example of the population: Little Albert was a typical child for his age and didn't have any characteristic that made him unique, while Peter had a phobia of white rats.

Some clinical practitioners use the single-case design to formally document clinical therapies of individual patients. Then they can submit the findings for further clinical investigation and evaluation.

My Experiment with Aroma-Conditioning

My experiment with aroma-conditioning also has the single-case design. The study participant has characteristics typical of a particular group —people with migraines.

Valid Argument for Aroma-Conditioning

Watson and Jones didn't have the opportunity to see the long term effects of Little Albert and Peter experiments. The researchers were forced by circumstances to discontinue their work. If I never have had another headache, my research would have been a single-case clinical study with an AB design, with the A standing for the initial assessment phase, and B the treatment phase.

With the AB design, I would surely have a clinical researcher, after reading my book, comment, "Your headaches might have disappeared as part of the natural course of your illness and there's no way to prove that your aroma-conditioning worked or that the therapy exists at all." These are good points because people suffering from chronic pain do have periods when pain appears more often and is felt more intensely. For a patient who has just received therapy and feels better, it's not important exactly how the therapy worked or if it had anything to do with the improvement. But for science, for clinical researchers, and for other patients, it is.

Because an AB design is less conclusive, if it's possible, a clinical researcher would design a single-case study that has more than one A and one B phase. An ABAB design is more likely than an AB design to prove a relationship between a treatment and improvement (or the independent and the dependent variables). Similarly, an ABABAB will produce more valid results than an ABAB and so on. The problem is that, in most cases, it is unethical to discontinue medical treatment if the patient or study participant feels better.

As a migraine patient, I didn't care about how scientific my treatment was as long as it worked. I just wanted my migraine headaches to stop. And I wouldn't discontinue my treatment so that it had scientific validity. But because my conditioned response (peppermint oil preventing headache phases of migraines) tended to wear off, I underwent two more A and B phases against my will. The scientist in me, however, was happy when writing this book, because the new phases further proved my hypothesis and ideas. (See Figure 10).

90

Figure 10
Aroma-Conditioning Experiment Turned Into Successful Treatment

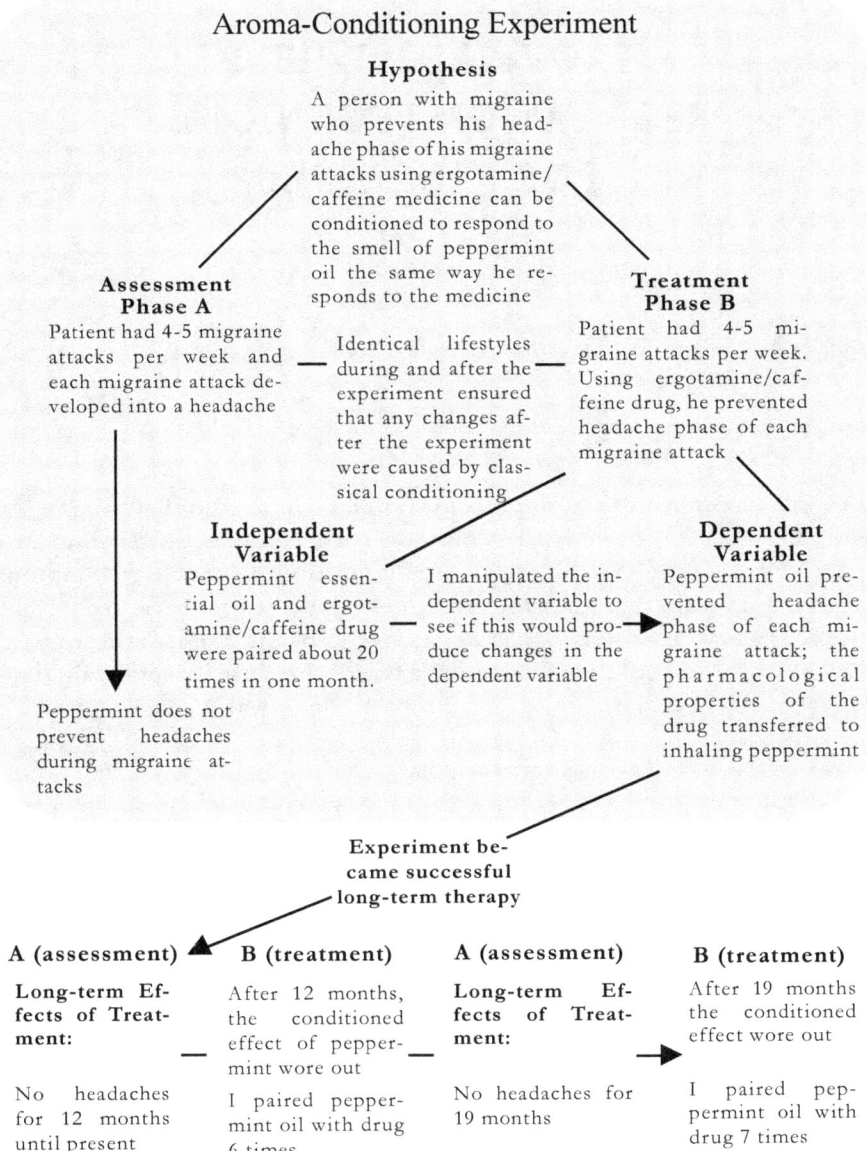

Aroma-Conditioning Experiment

Hypothesis

A person with migraine who prevents his headache phase of his migraine attacks using ergotamine/caffeine medicine can be conditioned to respond to the smell of peppermint oil the same way he responds to the medicine

Assessment Phase A

Patient had 4-5 migraine attacks per week and each migraine attack developed into a headache

Identical lifestyles during and after the experiment ensured that any changes after the experiment were caused by classical conditioning

Treatment Phase B

Patient had 4-5 migraine attacks per week. Using ergotamine/caffeine drug, he prevented headache phase of each migraine attack

Independent Variable

Peppermint essential oil and ergotamine/caffeine drug were paired about 20 times in one month.

I manipulated the independent variable to see if this would produce changes in the dependent variable

Dependent Variable

Peppermint oil prevented headache phase of each migraine attack; the pharmacological properties of the drug transferred to inhaling peppermint

Peppermint does not prevent headaches during migraine attacks

Experiment became successful long-term therapy

A (assessment)

Long-term Effects of Treatment:

No headaches for 12 months until present

B (treatment)

After 12 months, the conditioned effect of peppermint wore out

I paired peppermint oil with drug 6 times

A (assessment)

Long-term Effects of Treatment:

No headaches for 19 months

B (treatment)

After 19 months the conditioned effect wore out

I paired peppermint oil with drug 7 times

91

APPENDIX A

PROVEN SELF-HELP
RELAXATION TECHNIQUES
FOR MIGRAINES

As I was researching material for this book, I discovered that progressive muscle relaxation has a lot in common with aroma-conditioning. Progressive muscle relaxation and aroma-conditioning are both symptom-relieving, natural therapies for migraines. I decided to learn progressive muscle relaxation to see if it was effective in cutting short migraines. If it wasn't for the book, I wouldn't have tried it because it seemed difficult to learn. I also didn't think it would work. But I was wrong.

I was far from doing it right, from the first time—I contracted a number of muscles groups together with the targeted muscle. The third time I used progressive muscle relaxation at the first signs of preheadache, the symptoms went away faster than if I had used only peppermint oil. But there was more. The progressive muscle relaxation transformed the way I felt, from preheadache into a completely relaxed, physical and psychological well-being. This started to happen even though I had only gone through half my muscles.

Progressive muscle relaxation and the easiest breathing technique, the Slowing Down Respiration, can be combined during a migraine attack for greater effect. Both progressive muscle relaxation and the Slowing Down Respiration are relaxation techniques. These techniques are known to cut short migraine attacks, reduce pain, and when used daily, may even work as preventive therapy for migraines. The reason relaxation techniques work for migraines is that they reduce anxiety and promote relaxation. Anxiety and stress are common migraine triggers.

Breathing is an important part of aroma-conditioning, so it makes sense to learn some effective and easy breathing technique to use while inhaling the essential oil. Breathing techniques help manage migraine pain, because when you are under stress, your heart rate and breathing become rapid. This increases the blood flow to your muscles and your brain becomes more sensitive. Breathing techniques help you lower your heart rate, by slowing your breathing. This helps you relax.

Slowing Down Respiration

The Slowing Down Respiration Technique is the easiest to learn and one of the most effective breathing techniques. It can be practiced while sitting or walking. The purpose of the technique is to reduce rapid breathing to 10-12 breaths per minute, which is the normal breathing rate for most adults.

1. Place one hand over the lower part of your ribs, above your stomach. Feel your hand moving in and out as you inhale and exhale. Try not to move your shoulders while breathing.

2. Inhale deeply and slowly through your nose, with your mouth closed; exhale though your mouth. Both breathing in and out must take about 3 seconds each.

3. Keep with this exercise until your breathing rate reaches 10-12 breaths per minute.

Progressive Muscle Relaxation

Progressive muscle relaxation (PMR) is a technique used in anxiety and stress management. It was developed by American psychologist Edmund Jacobson in 1929. When mastered, the therapy leads to deep muscle relaxation, which reduces physiological tension, lowers the heart rate and blood pressure, and slows breathing. Progressive muscle relaxation is widely-used today because it has been an effective remedy for treating various disorders—muscle tension, insomnia, fatigue, depression, high-blood pressure, neck and back pain, stuttering, phobias, and muscle spasms. The technique involves tensing muscles and muscle groups and relaxing them in succession.

How to Begin

You can practice progressive muscle relaxation sitting on a chair with your head supported or lying on your back. When lying on your back, keep your eyes closed, arms away from your sides, palms upward, and legs slightly apart.

Start with inhaling deeply and slowly through your nose. Exhale through your mouth and repeat several times. You may use the Slowing Down Respiration technique.

How to Tense Your Muscles

The technique is the same for all muscles: focus your mind on the muscle, take a deep breath, and tense the muscle. Hold for 5-8 seconds. You must tense as hard as you can, until your it becomes painful and your muscle starts shaking. The muscles of the neck, back, toes, and feet must not be tensed too much or you may injure yourself.

Now release the muscle at once and let it relax. Breath out, imagining the tension flowing away from the muscle and from the muscles you worked before that. Relax for 15-20 seconds before you start working the next muscle group.

You must focus completely on the muscle relaxation and try to feel the difference between tensed and relaxed muscles. Try to do this for every separate muscle.

Beginners tend to tense other muscles groups together with the targeted muscle group. This is normal. With practice, you will learn how to tense only one muscle group at a time. The more you practice, the better you'll become.

Muscles Sequence

Experts say that the best practice is to start working your muscles from your feet up. But I found that during a migraine attack, the technique is more effective to start from your head down. Experiment and find what is more effective for you.

Right calf and foot: Point toes, tense for 8 seconds; relax. (Don't raise your leg);

Right thigh: Extend and raise leg about 6 inches, tense for 8 seconds; relax;

Entire right leg:: Point toes and raise leg about 6 inches, tense calf, foot, and thigh; relax;

Left calf and foot;

Left thigh;

Entire left leg;

Right hand and forearm: Clench your fist tightly and tense forearm and hand muscles for 8 seconds; relax;

Right bicep and triceps: Bend your elbow and tense your bicep; relax. Extend your arm and tense your triceps; relax;

Entire right arm: Clench your fist tightly and tense forearm, bicep, and triceps; relax;

Left hand and forearm;

Left bicep and triceps;

Entire left arm;

Buttocks: Raise your pelvis a little and tense; relax;

Stomach: Tense stomach; relax;

Back: Arch your upper body forward, pushing your shoulders backward, and tense your back muscles; relax;

Chest: Tense chest muscles; relax;

Shoulders: Pull your shoulders up toward your ears and tense; relax;

Neck: With the shoulders relaxed and leveled, push your chin toward your chest and tense; relax;

Mouth: Gape as wide as possible and tense the muscles around your mouth; relax;

Lips: Purse your lips as tight as possible and tense; relax;

Tongue: With your mouth open, extend your tongue as far as possible and tense for 8 seconds; relax for 20 seconds; take your tongue back into your mouth and push it as far back as possible; tense for 8 seconds; relax for 20;

Eyes: Open your eyes wrinkling your forehead as tight as possible; relax. Squeeze your eyes as tight as you can; relax.

After you finish, spend a couple of minutes with your eyes closed. If you've completed it correctly, your whole body will feel light and completely relaxed.

APPENDIX B

SELF-EFFICACY

Sense of Self-Efficacy and Achievement

Sense of self-efficacy, also known as perceived self-efficacy, is your belief that you can successfully finish tasks and accomplish goals. People with high self-efficacy are likely to make greater effort over longer period of time, despite difficulties. Such people view difficult tasks as challenges that can be overcome through learning and experience; they regain their sense of self-efficacy shortly after a failure, and they attribute failure to insufficient effort—not to lack of ability. Thus, "a strong sense of self-efficacy enhances human accomplishment and personal well-being in many ways" (Bandura, 1994).

Low self-efficacy, on the other hand, can make people believe that things are more difficult than they really are. People with low self-efficacy give up easily, have "weak commitment

Emotional and Intellectual Self-Efficacy?

Psychologists A.A. Sappington and J.C. Russell suggest that there are two more kinds of expectations that can predict people's behavior—intellectually based and emotionally based. The researchers say that emotional expectations come from our emotional reactions to things, not from logical thinking. Thus, a distinction must be made between emotional and intellectual self-efficacy.

97

to goals," are slow in recovering from failure, prone to "stress and depression," and likely to attribute failure to lack of ability on their side—rather than lack of effort and commitment (Bandura, 1994).

Self-Efficacy and Motivation

In psychology, motivation can be defined as the level of willingness or eagerness to achieve goals or, simply, how much do you want to achieve something and the effort you are willing put into achieving it. And a strong sense of self-efficacy can greatly influence strong motivation. "Self-efficacy beliefs contribute to motivation in several ways: They determine the goals people set for themselves; how much effort they expend; how long they persevere in the face of difficulties; and their resilience to failures" (Bandura, 1994).

Self-Efficacy, Motivation, Medical Treatment, and Healthy Lifestyle

In medical settings, a patient's level of self-efficacy and motivation predict not only how active he or she will be in a treatment—which directly influences the outcome of the treatment—but also whether the patient will actually do something about their medical problem. And all general benefits of strong self-efficacy and strong motivation apply to medical treatment. A motivated person with strong self-efficacy beliefs will make any medical treatment more successful—he or she will persist longer, will not be discouraged by difficulties, and put a lot of effort.

Strong self-efficacy can also promote a healthy lifestyle—a person with a strong self-efficacy who decides to lead a healthier lifestyle is more likely to succeed because he or she will not give up easily when working on his or her healthy goals.

Self-Efficacy, Anxiety, and Stress

Anxiety and stress, in addition to being common migraine triggers, can lead to physical illnesses. For example, there is scientific evidence showing that stress and anxiety weaken the immune system, and a weak immune system cannot protect the body from infection caused by invading organisms and toxic substances, which can lead to various diseases. People with low sense of self-efficacy are less able to cope with stressful situations, and thus may become susceptible to illness; Albert Bandura says that "it is not stressful life conditions per se, but the perceived inability to manage them that is debilitating."

APPENDIX C

QUESTIONNAIRES TO MEASURE YOUR EXPECTATIONS

	Agree Strongly	Agree	Neither Agree Nor Disagree	Disagree	Disagree Strongly

General Self-Efficacy Expectancies

I am certain I can accomplish the goals I have in life.

	Agree Strongly	Agree	Neither Agree Nor Disagree	Disagree	Disagree Strongly
Just before the therapy			X		
3 month after therapy started			X		
3 years after therapy started	X				

I view difficulties as challenges and I never give up.

	Agree Strongly	Agree	Neither Agree Nor Disagree	Disagree	Disagree Strongly
Just before the therapy		X			
3 month after therapy started		X			
3 years after therapy started		X			

I attribute my failures to lack of effort and external difficulties.

	Agree Strongly	Agree	Neither Agree Nor Disagree	Disagree	Disagree Strongly
Just before the therapy		X			
3 month after therapy started		X			
3 years after therapy started		X			

Figure 11
My General Self-Efficacy Expectancies before, during, and after Aroma-Conditioning

Outcome Expectancies

I believe that Western science and medicine are effective and true.

	Agree Strongly	Agree	Neither Agree Nor Disagree	Disagree	Disagree Strongly
Just before the therapy	X				
3 month after therapy started	X				
3 years after therapy started	X				

I believe that, in general, classical conditioning is effective for migraine.

	Agree Strongly	Agree	Neither Agree Nor Disagree	Disagree	Disagree Strongly
Just before the therapy			X		
3 month after therapy started	X				
3 years after therapy started	X				

I believe that ergotamine is an effective medicine for migraine headaches.

	Agree Strongly	Agree	Neither Agree Nor Disagree	Disagree	Disagree Strongly
Just before the therapy		X			
3 month after therapy started	X				
3 years after therapy started	X				

I believe that peppermint oil has a natural properties that relieve migraine headaches.

	Agree Strongly	Agree	Neither Agree Nor Disagree	Disagree	Disagree Strongly
Just before the therapy		X			
3 month after therapy started		X			
3 years after therapy started	X				

Self-Efficacy Expectancies

I am certain that aroma-conditioning prevents migraine headaches.

	Agree Strongly	Agree	Neither Agree Nor Disagree	Disagree	Disagree Strongly
Just before the therapy			X		
3 month after therapy started		X			
3 years after therapy started	X				

I am certain I'm in control of my migraine.

	Agree Strongly	Agree	Neither Agree Nor Disagree	Disagree	Disagree Strongly
Just before the therapy					X
3 month after therapy started		X			
3 years after therapy started	X				

Figure 12

My Outcome and Self-Efficacy Expectancies before, during, and after Aroma-Conditioning

JONES'S EXPERIMENT
WITH PETER VS.
MY AROMA-CONDITIONING
EXPERIMENT

Making Sure You Treat What You Should

Jones's experiment and mine both have the single-case design. Her main hypothesis was that unreasonable fear of a child can be counter- conditioned or reversed by classical conditioning. For her study Jones selected Peter, because he was a typical, healthy child who "was well adjusted except for his exaggerated fear reactions" (Jones, 1924, p. 462). These characteristics of Peter ensured Jones that her findings would apply to children with phobia in general.

In my experiment, I used one participant who, except for his migraine headaches, is healthy and typical of the population, overall. This made my findings apply to people with migraine in general. But with my experiment, I wanted to achieve the opposite of what Jones's intended: instead of extinguishing a conditioned response, I wanted to create one. I wanted to get the mint oil work the same way as the drug.

Controlling Your Experiment

Jones tried to control, as much as possible, all other aspects of her experiment besides the treatment. For example, she did her experiment in a laboratory, where she was able to eliminate external influences. I controlled my experiment by keeping everything constant except the treatment, to make sure that changes in the dependent variable—the results of peppermint oil serving as medicine—were actually caused by the treatment, and not from something else. That is, except for using aroma-conditioning, I did not change anything else in my lifestyle.

Assessment Phase (A Phase)

Jones began her study with initial assessment of Peter. First, she made sure that Peter is a child that in fact had the unreasonable fear she wanted to remove: "At sight of the rat, Peter screamed and fell flat on his back" (Jones, 1924, p. 463). She also studied Peter's other personality traits—how he behaved among other children and adults, and how he adjusted, and she even gave him an IQ test. This part of the clinical single-case design, where the researcher studies the participant or patient, is known as the baseline phase or A. During this phase, the researcher identifies the general pattern of symptoms, and findings are compared to the results of the next phase—treatment phase or B.

In Chapter VII, "Migraine, Drugs, and Aromatherapy," I describe the study participant in my experiment. His personality, background, and the history of his migraine. I identify the pattern of migraine symptoms just before the treatment phase with aroma-conditioning, and compare those symptoms after the treatment phase.

Treatment Phase (B Phase)

During the treatment phase, Peter underwent a series classical conditioning pairings: white rabbit with candy and other children playing with rabbit. Jones's independent variable was the treatment—counter-conditioning, a form of classical conditioning, which she measured by the number of pairings. The main dependent variable was fear that Peter felt at different degrees, at different stages during the treatment phase.

My participant also went through a series of classical conditioning trials. (See Chapter VIII, "Aroma-Conditioning in Action.") My independent variable was the treatment with classical conditioning. The dependent variable was peppermint oil preventing headaches.

Findings

After the treatment, Jones was certain that Peter's fear was gone; she compared the initial reaction of fear with the Peter's eventual affection toward the white rabbit—"fondles rabbit affectionately" (Jones, 1924, p. 465). So, Jones's hypothesis of the study was confirmed—that phobias can be extinguished using counterconditioning.

After my treatment with aroma-conditioning, peppermint oil alone prevented headaches. And my hypothesis was confirmed more than once. To see how my hypothesis was confirmed and why the treatment was successful, see Chapter IV, "Aroma-Conditioning in Action."

REFERENCES

Amanzio, M. & Benedetti, F. (1999). Neuropharmacological dissection of placebo analgesia: expectation-activated opioid systems versus conditioning-activated specific subsystems. *J Neurosci, 19*(1), 484–494. Retrieved July 30, 2009, from http://www.ncbi.nlm.nih.gov/pubmed/9870976

American Council for Headache Education (with Constantine, L. M. & Scott, S.). (1994). *Migraine: The complete guide.* New York: Dell Pub.

Bandura, A. (1994). Self-efficacy. In V. S. Ramachaudran (Ed.), *Encyclopedia of human behavior* (Vol. 4, pp. 71-81). New York: Academic Press. (Reprinted in H. Friedman [Ed.], *Encyclopedia of mental health.* San Diego: Academic Press, 1998). Retrieved June 22, 2009, from http://www.des.emory.edu/mfp/BanEncy.html

Benedetti, F. (2006, May 3). Placebo analgesia. *Neurological Sciences, 27,* s100-s102. Retrieved November 26, 2008, from EBSCOhost database.

Crow, R., Gage, H., Hampson, S., Hart, J., Kimber, A. & Thomas, H. (1999). The role of expectancies in the placebo effect and their use in the delivery of health care: a systematic review. *Health Technology Assess-*

ment, 3(3). Retrieved November 12, 2008, from http://www.ncchta.org/execsumm/summ303.htm

Diamond, M. (2007). The impact of migraine on the health and well-being of women. *Journal of Women's Health, 16*(9), 1269-1280. Retrieved February 15, 2008, from EBSCOhost database.

Hawkins, K., Rupnow, M. & Wang, S. (April 2008) Direct cost burden among insured US employees with migraine. *The Journal of Head & Face Pain, 48*(4), 553-563. Retrieved July 2, 2009, from EBSCOhost database.

International Journal of Toxicology. (2001). Final report on the safety assessment of Mentha Piperita (peppermint) oil, Mentha Piperita (peppermint) leaf extract, Mentha Piperita (peppermint) leaf, and Mentha Piperita (peppermint) leaf water. *20*, 61-73. Retrieved April 9, 2008, from EBSCOhost database.

Jones, M. C. (1924). A laboratory study of fear: The case of Peter. *Journal of Genetic Psychology, 152*(4), 462. Retriever December 1, 2007, from EBSCOhost database.

Koshi, E., Short, C. (March, 2007). Placebo theory and its implications for research and clinical practice: a review of the recent literature. *Pain Practice, 7*(1), 4-20. Retrieved December 3, 2008, from EBSCOhost database.

McCaleb, R. (1995). Essential oils for fast relief of headache pain. *HerbalGram, 35*, 12-12. Retrieved April 11, 2008, from EBSCOhost database.

Mikalsen, A., Bertelsen, B., & Flaten, M. (2001, October). Effects of caffeine, caffeine-associated stimuli, and caffeine-related information on physiological and psychological arousal. Psychopharmacology, 157(4), 373-380. Retrieved August 18, 2009, from MEDLINE with Full Text database.

Stewart-Williams, S. & Podd, J. (March, 2004). The placebo effect: Dissolving the expectancy versus conditioning debate. *Psychological Bulletin, 130*(2), 324-340. Retrieved November 18, 2008, from EBSCOhost database.

Watson, J. B. (1930). *Behaviorism* (revised edition). Chicago: University of Chicago Press.

Watson, J. B. & Rayner, R. (1920). Conditioned emotional reactions. *American Psychologist, 55*(3), 313-317. Retrieved November 30, 2007, from EBSCOhost database.